PALEO COOKBOOK 2022

TASTY RECIPES FOR BEGINNERS

JEREMY BUSH

Table of Contents

Grilled Strip Steaks with Grated Root Vegetable Hash 10
Asian Beef and Vegetable Stir-Fry 12
Cedar-Planked Filets with Asian Slather and Slaw 14
Pan-Seared Tri-Tip Steaks with Cauliflower Peperonata 17
Flat-Iron Steaks au Poivre with Mushroom-Dijon Sauce 19
Steaks 19
Sauce 19
Grilled Flat-Iron Steaks with Chipotle-Caramelized Onions and Salsa Salad 22
Steaks 22
Salsa Salad 22
Caramelized Onions 22
Grilled Ribeyes with Herbed Onion and Garlic "Butter" 25
Ribeye Salad with Grilled Beets 27
Korean-Style Short Ribs with Sautéed Ginger Cabbage 29
Beef Short Ribs with Citrus-Fennel Gremolata 32
Ribs 32
Pan-Roasted Squash 32
Gremolata 32
Swedish-Style Beef Patties with Mustard-Dill Cucumber Salad 35
Cucumber Salad 35
Beef Patties 35
Smothered Beefburgers on Arugula with Roasted Root Vegetables 39
Grilled Beefburgers with Sesame-Crusted Tomatoes 42
Burgers on a Stick with Baba Ghanoush Dipping Sauce 44
Smoky Stuffed Sweet Peppers 46
Bison Burgers with Cabernet Onions and Arugula 48
Bison and Lamb Meat Loaf on Chard and Sweet Potatoes 51
Apple-Currant-Sauced Bison Meatballs with Zucchini Pappardelle 54
Meatballs 54
Apple-Currant Sauce 54
Zucchini Pappardelle 54

Bison-Porcini Bolognese with Roasted Garlic Spaghetti Squash 57
Bison Chili con Carne 59
Moroccan-Spiced Bison Steaks with Grilled Lemons 61
Herbes de Provence-Rubbed Bison Sirloin Roast 62
Coffee-Braised Bison Short Ribs with Tangerine Gremolata and Celery Root Mash 64
Marinade 64
Braise 64
Beef Bone Broth 67
Tunisian Spice-Rubbed Pork Shoulder with Spicy Sweet Potato Fries 69
Pork 69
Fries 69
Cuban Grilled Pork Shoulder 71
Italian Spice-Rubbed Pork Roast with Vegetables 74
Slow Cooker Pork Mole 76
Caraway-Spiced Pork and Squash Stew 78
Fruit-Stuffed Top Loin Roast with Brandy Sauce 80
Roast 80
Brandy Sauce 80
Porchetta-Style Pork Roast 83
Tomatillo-Braised Pork Loin 85
Apricot-Stuffed Pork Tenderloin 87
Herb-Crusted Pork Tenderloin with Crispy Garlic Oil 89
Indian-Spiced Pork with Coconut Pan Sauce 90
Pork Scaloppini with Spiced Apples and Chestnuts 91
Pork Fajita Stir-Fry 94
Pork Tenderloin with Port and Prunes 95
Moo Shu-Style Pork in Lettuce Cups with Quick Pickled Vegetables 97
Pickled Vegetables 97
Pork 97
Pork Chops with Macadamias, Sage, Figs, and Mashed Sweet Potatoes ... 99
Skillet-Roasted Rosemary-Lavender Pork Chops with Grapes and Toasted Walnuts
 101
Pork Chops alla Fiorentina with Grilled Broccoli Rabe 103
Escarole-Stuffed Pork Chops 105
Pork Chops with a Dijon-Pecan Crust 108

Walnut-Crusted Pork with Blackberry Spinach Salad ... 109

Pork Schnitzel with Sweet-and-Sour Red Cabbage ... 111

Cabbage ... 111

Pork 111

Roasted Turkey with Garlicky Mashed Roots ... 113

Stuffed Turkey Breast with Pesto Sauce and Arugula Salad ... 115

Spiced Turkey Breast with Cherry BBQ Sauce ... 117

Wine-Braised Turkey Tenderloin ... 119

Pan-Sautéed Turkey Breast with Chive Scampi Sauce ... 122

Braised Turkey Legs with Root Vegetables ... 124

Herbed Turkey Meat Loaf with Caramelized Onion Ketchup and Roasted Cabbage Wedges ... 126

Turkey Posole ... 128

Chicken Bone Broth ... 130

Green Harissa Salmon ... 133

Salmon ... 133

Harissa ... 133

Spiced Sunflower Seeds ... 133

Salad 133

Grilled Salmon with Marinated Artichoke Heart Salad ... 136

Flash-Roasted Chile-Sage Salmon with Green Tomato Salsa ... 138

Salmon ... 138

Green Tomato Salsa ... 138

Roasted Salmon and Asparagus en Papillote with Lemon-Hazelnut Pesto ... 140

Spice-Rubbed Salmon with Mushroom-Apple Pan Sauce ... 142

Sole en Papillote with Julienne Vegetables ... 145

Arugula Pesto Fish Tacos with Smoky Lime Cream ... 147

Almond-Crusted Sole ... 149

Grilled Cod and Zucchini Packets with Spicy Mango-Basil Sauce ... 151

Riesling-Poached Cod with Pesto-Stuffed Tomatoes ... 153

Broiled Pistachio-Cilantro-Crusted Cod over Smashed Sweet Potatoes ... 155

Rosemary-and-Tangerine Cod with Roasted Broccoli ... 157

Curried Cod Lettuce Wraps with Pickled Radishes ... 159

Roasted Haddock with Lemon and Fennel ... 161

Pecan-Crusted Snapper with Remoulade and Cajun-Style Okra and Tomatoes ... 163

Tarragon Tuna Patties with Avocado-Lemon Aïoli 165
Striped Bass Tagine 168
Halibut in Garlic-Shrimp Sauce with Soffrito Collard Greens 170
Seafood Bouillabaisse 172
Classic Shrimp Ceviche 174
Coconut-Crusted Shrimp and Spinach Salad 177
Tropical Shrimp and Scallop Ceviche 179
Jamaican Jerk Shrimp with Avocado Oil 181
Shrimp Scampi with Wilted Spinach and Radicchio 182
Crab Salad with Avocado, Grapefruit, and Jicama 184
Cajun Lobster Tail Boil with Tarragon Aïoli 186
Mussels Frites with Saffron Aïoli 188
Parsnip Frites 188
Saffron Aïoli 188
Mussels 188
Seared Scallops with Beet Relish 191
Grilled Scallops with Cucumber-Dill Salsa 193
Seared Scallops with Tomato, Olive Oil, and Herb Sauce 195
Scallops and Sauce 195
Salad 195
Cumin-Roasted Cauliflower with Fennel and Pearl Onions 197
Chunky Tomato-Eggplant Sauce with Spaghetti Squash 199
Stuffed Portobello Mushrooms 201
Roasted Radicchio 203
Roasted Fennel with Orange Vinaigrette 204
Punjabi-Style Savoy Cabbage 207
Cinnamon-Roasted Butternut Squash 209
Broiled Asparagus with Sieved Egg and Pecans 210
Crunchy Cabbage Slaw with Radishes, Mango, and Mint 212
Roasted Cabbage Rounds with Caraway and Lemon 213
Roasted Cabbage with Orange-Balsamic Drizzle 214
Braised Cabbage with Creamy Dill Sauce and Toasted Walnuts 215
Sautéed Green Cabbage with Toasted Sesame Seeds 216

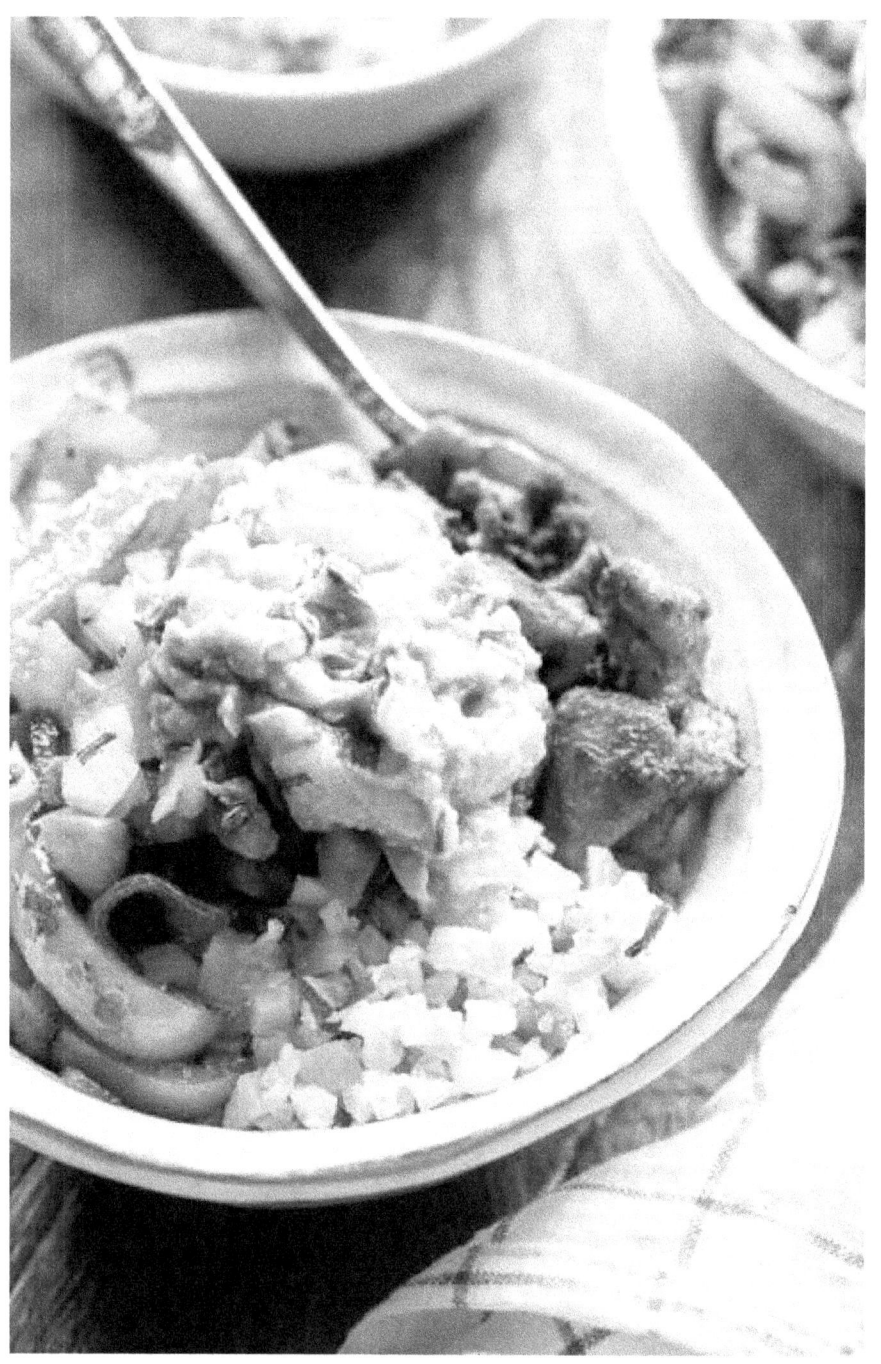

GRILLED STRIP STEAKS WITH GRATED ROOT VEGETABLE HASH

PREP: 20 minutes STAND: 20 minutes GRILL: 10 minutes STAND: 5 minutes MAKES: 4 servings

STRIP STEAKS HAVE A VERY TENDER TEXTURE, AND THE SMALL STRIP OF FAT ON ONE SIDE OF THE STEAK GETS CRISP AND SMOKY ON THE GRILL. MY THINKING ABOUT ANIMAL FAT HAS CHANGED SINCE MY FIRST BOOK. IF YOU ARE FAITHFUL TO THE BASIC PRINCIPLES OF THE PALEO DIET® AND KEEP SATURATED FATS WITHIN 10 TO 15 PERCENT OF YOUR DAILY CALORIES, IT WILL NOT INCREASE YOUR RISK OF HEART DISEASE—AND IN FACT, THE OPPOSITE MAY BE TRUE. NEW INFORMATION SUGGESTS THAT ELEVATIONS IN LDL CHOLESTEROL MAY ACTUALLY REDUCE SYSTEMIC INFLAMMATION, WHICH IS A RISK FACTOR FOR HEART DISEASE.

3 tablespoons extra virgin olive oil

2 tablespoons grated fresh horseradish

1 teaspoon finely shredded orange peel

½ teaspoon ground cumin

½ teaspoon black pepper

4 strip steaks (also called top loin), cut about 1 inch thick

2 medium parsnips, peeled

1 large sweet potato, peeled

1 medium turnip, peeled

1 or 2 shallots, finely chopped

2 cloves garlic, minced

1 tablespoon snipped fresh thyme

1. In a small bowl stir together 1 tablespoon of the oil, horseradish, orange peel, cumin, and ¼ teaspoon of the

pepper. Spread the mixture over steaks; cover and let stand at room temperature for 15 minutes.

2. Meanwhile for hash, using a box grater or a food processor fitted with the shredding blade, shred the parsnips, sweet potato, and turnip. Place shredded vegetables in a large bowl; add shallot(s). In a small bowl combine the remaining 2 tablespoons oil, the remaining ¼ teaspoon pepper, garlic, and thyme. Drizzle over vegetables; toss to mix thoroughly. Fold a 36×18-inch piece of heavy foil in half to make a double thickness of foil that measures 18×18 inches. Place vegetable mixture in the center of the foil; bring up opposite edges of foil and seal with a double fold. Fold remaining edges to completely enclose the vegetables, leaving space for steam to build.

3. For a charcoal or gas grill, place steaks and foil packet on the grill rack directly over medium heat. Cover and grill steaks for 10 to 12 minutes for medium rare (145°F) or 12 to 15 minutes for medium (160°F), turning once halfway through grilling. Grill packet for 10 to 15 minutes or until vegetables are tender. Let steaks stand for 5 minutes while vegetables finish cooking. Divide vegetable hash among four serving plates; top with steaks.

ASIAN BEEF AND VEGETABLE STIR-FRY

PREP: 30 minutes COOK: 15 minutes MAKES: 4 servings

FIVE-SPICE POWDER IS A SALT-FREE SPICE BLEND USED WIDELY IN CHINESE COOKING. IT CONSISTS OF EQUAL PARTS GROUND CINNAMON, CLOVES, FENNEL SEEDS, STAR ANISE, AND SZECHWAN PEPPERCORNS.

- 1½ pounds boneless beef top sirloin steak or boneless beef round steak, cut 1 inch thick
- 1½ teaspoons five-spice powder
- 3 tablespoons refined coconut oil
- 1 small red onion, cut into thin wedges
- 1 small bunch asparagus (about 12 ounces), trimmed and cut into 3-inch pieces
- 1½ cups julienne-cut orange and/or yellow carrots
- 4 cloves garlic, minced
- 1 teaspoon finely shredded orange peel
- ¼ cup fresh orange juice
- ¼ cup Beef Bone Broth (see recipe) or no-salt-added beef broth
- ¼ cup white wine vinegar
- ¼ to ½ teaspoon crushed red pepper
- 8 cups coarsely shredded napa cabbage
- ½ cup unsalted slivered almonds or unsalted coarsely chopped cashews, toasted (see tip, page 57)

1. If desired, partially freeze beef for easier slicing (about 20 minutes). Cut beef into very thin slices. In a large bowl toss together beef and five-spice powder. In a large wok or extra-large skillet heat 1 tablespoon of the coconut oil over medium-high heat. Add half the beef; cook and stir for 3 to 5 minutes or until browned. Transfer beef to a bowl. Repeat with the remaining beef and another 1

tablespoon oil. Transfer beef to the bowl with the other cooked beef.

2. In the same wok add the remaining 1 tablespoon oil. Add onion; cook and stir for 3 minutes. Add asparagus and carrots; cook and stir for 2 to 3 minutes or until vegetables are crisp-tender. Add garlic; cook and stir for 1 minute more.

3. For sauce, in a small bowl combine orange peel, orange juice, Beef Bone Broth, vinegar, and crushed red pepper. Add sauce and all the beef with juices in bowl to vegetables in wok. Cook and stir for 1 to 2 minutes or until heated through. Using a slotted spoon, transfer beef vegetables to a large bowl. Cover to keep warm.

4. Cook the sauce, uncovered, over medium heat for 2 minutes. Add cabbage; cook and stir for 1 to 2 minutes or until cabbage is just wilted. Divide cabbage and any cooking juices among four serving plates. Top evenly with beef mixture. Sprinkle with nuts.

CEDAR-PLANKED FILETS WITH ASIAN SLATHER AND SLAW

SOAK: 1 hour PREP: 40 minutes GRILL: 13 minutes STAND: 10 minutes MAKES: 4 servings.

NAPA CABBAGE IS SOMETIMES CALLED CHINESE CABBAGE. IT HAS BEAUTIFUL, CRINKLY CREAM-COLOR LEAVES WITH BRIGHT YELLOW-GREEN TIPS. IT HAS A DELICATE, MILD FLAVOR AND TEXTURE—QUITE DIFFERENT THAN THE WAXY LEAVES OF ROUND-HEADED CABBAGE—AND NOT SURPRISINGLY, IS A NATURAL IN ASIAN-STYLE DISHES.

1 large cedar plank
¼ ounce dried shiitake mushrooms
¼ cup walnut oil
2 teaspoons minced fresh ginger
2 teaspoons crushed red pepper
1 teaspoon crushed Szechwan peppercorns
¼ teaspoon five-spice powder
4 cloves garlic, minced
4 4- to 5-ounce beef tenderloin steaks, cut ¾ to 1 inch thick
Asian Slaw (see recipe, below)

1. Place grill plank in water; weight down and soak for at least 1 hour.

2. Meanwhile, for Asian slather, in a small bowl pour boiling water over dried shiitake mushrooms; let stand for 20 minutes to rehydrate. Drain mushrooms and place in a food processor. Add walnut oil, ginger, crushed red pepper, Szechuan peppercorns, five-spice powder, and garlic. Cover and process until mushrooms are minced and ingredients are combined; set aside.

3. Drain grill plank. For a charcoal grill, arrange medium-hot coals around perimeter of grill. Place plank on grill rack directly over coals. Cover and grill for 3 to 5 minutes or until plank begins to crackle and smoke. Place steaks on grill rack directly over coals; grill for 3 to 4 minutes or until seared. Transfer steaks to the plank, seared sides up. Place plank in center of grill. Divide Asian Slather among steaks. Cover and grill for 10 to 12 minutes or until an instant-read thermometer inserted horizontally into the steaks reads 130°F. (For a gas grill, preheat grill. Reduce heat to medium. Place drained plank on grill rack; cover and grill for 3 to 5 minutes or until plank begins to crackle and smoke. Place steaks on grill rack for 3 to 4 minutes or until seared. Transfer steaks to the plank, seared sides up. Adjust grill for indirect cooking; place plank with steaks over the burner that is turned off. Divide slather among steaks. Cover and grill for 10 to 12 minutes or until an instant-read thermometer inserted horizontally into the steaks reads 130°F.)

4. Remove steaks from the grill. Cover steaks loosely with foil; let stand for 10 minutes. Cut steaks into ¼-inch-thick slices. Serve steak over Asian Slaw.

Asian Slaw: In a large bowl combine 1 medium head napa cabbage, thinly sliced; 1 cup finely shredded red cabbage; 2 carrots, peeled and cut into julienne strips; 1 red or yellow sweet pepper, seeded and very thinly sliced; 4 scallions, thinly bias-sliced; 1 to 2 serrano chiles, seeded and minced (see tip); 2 tablespoons chopped cilantro; and 2 tablespoons chopped mint. For dressing, in a food processor or blender combine 3 tablespoons fresh lime juice, 1 tablespoon grated fresh ginger, 1 cloves minced garlic, and ⅛ teaspoon five-spice powder. Cover and process until smooth. With the processor running, gradually add ½ cup walnut oil and process until smooth. Add 1 scallion, thinly bias-sliced, to the dressing. Drizzle over slaw and toss to coat.

PAN-SEARED TRI-TIP STEAKS WITH CAULIFLOWER PEPERONATA

PREP: 25 minutes COOK: 25 minutes MAKES: 2 servings

PEPERONATA IS TRADITIONALLY A SLOW-ROASTED RAGU OF SWEET PEPPERS WITH ONION, GARLIC, AND HERBS. THIS QUICK SAUTÉED VERSION—MADE HEARTIER WITH CAULIFLOWER—ACTS AS BOTH RELISH AND SIDE DISH.

2 4- to 6-ounce tri-tip steaks, cut ¾ to 1 inch thick
¾ teaspoon black pepper
2 tablespoons extra virgin olive oil
2 red and/or yellow sweet peppers, seeded and sliced
1 shallot, thinly sliced
1 teaspoon Mediterranean Seasoning (see recipe)
2 cups small cauliflower florets
2 tablespoons balsamic vinegar
2 teaspoons snipped fresh thyme

1. Pat steaks dry with paper towels. Sprinkle steaks with ¼ teaspoon of the black pepper. In a large skillet heat 1 tablespoon of the oil over medium-high heat. Add steaks to skillet; reduce heat to medium. Cook steaks for 6 to 9 minutes for medium rare (145°F), turning occasionally. (If meat browns too quickly, reduce heat.) Remove steaks from skillet; cover loosely with foil to keep warm.

2. For the peperonata, add the remaining 1 tablespoon oil to the skillet. Add the sweet peppers and shallot. Sprinkle with Mediterranean Seasoning. Cook over medium heat about 5 minutes or until peppers are softened, stirring occasionally. Add cauliflower, balsamic vinegar, thyme,

and the remaining ½ teaspoon black pepper. Cover and cook for 10 to 15 minutes or until cauliflower is tender, stirring occasionally. Return steaks to skillet. Spoon peperonata mixture over steaks. Serve immediately.

FLAT-IRON STEAKS AU POIVRE WITH MUSHROOM-DIJON SAUCE

PREP: 15 minutes COOK: 20 minutes MAKES: 4 servings

THIS FRENCH-INSPIRED STEAK WITH MUSHROOM SAUCE CAN BE ON THE TABLE IN JUST OVER 30 MINUTES—WHICH MAKES IT A GREAT CHOICE FOR A QUICK WEEKNIGHT MEAL.

STEAKS
- 3 tablespoons extra virgin olive oil
- 1 pound small asparagus spears, trimmed
- 4 6-ounce flat-iron (boneless beef shoulder top blade) steaks*
- 2 tablespoons snipped fresh rosemary
- 1½ teaspoons cracked black pepper

SAUCE
- 8 ounces sliced fresh mushrooms
- 2 cloves garlic, minced
- ½ cup Beef Bone Broth (see recipe)
- ¼ cup dry white wine
- 1 tablespoon Dijon-Style Mustard (see recipe)

1. In a large skillet heat 1 tablespoon of the oil over medium-high heat. Add asparagus; cook for 8 to 10 minutes or until crisp-tender, turning spears occasionally so they don't burn. Transfer asparagus to a plate; cover with foil to keep warm.

2. Sprinkle steaks with rosemary and pepper; rub in with your fingers. In the same skillet heat the remaining 2 tablespoons oil over medium-high heat. Add steaks; reduce heat to medium. Cook for 8 to 12 minutes for medium rare (145°F), turning meat occasionally. (If meat

browns too quickly, reduce heat.) Remove meat from skillet, reserving drippings. Cover steaks loosely with foil to keep warm.

3. For sauce, add mushrooms and garlic to drippings in skillet; cook until tender, stirring occasionally. Add broth, wine, and Dijon-Style Mustard. Cook over medium heat, scraping up the browned bits in bottom of skillet. Bring to boiling; cook for 1 minute more.

4. Divide the asparagus among four dinner plates. Top with steaks; spoon sauce over the steaks.

*Note: If you can't find 6-ounce flat-iron steaks, purchase two 8- to 12-ounce steaks and cut them in half to make four steaks.

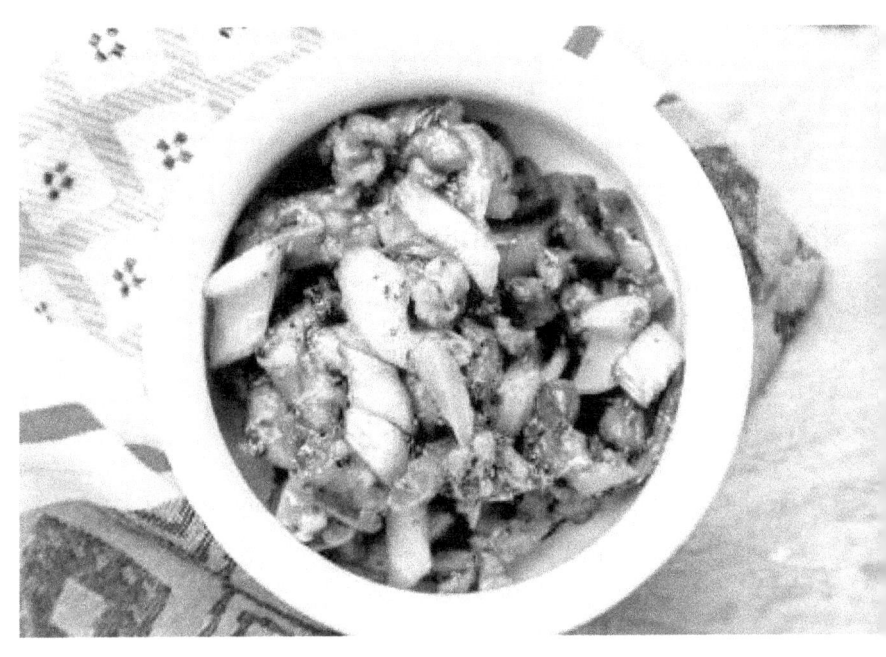

GRILLED FLAT-IRON STEAKS WITH CHIPOTLE-CARAMELIZED ONIONS AND SALSA SALAD

PREP: 30 minutes MARINATE: 2 hours BAKE: 20 minutes COOL: 20 minutes GRILL: 45 minutes MAKES: 4 servings

FLAT-IRON STEAK IS A RELATIVELY NEW CUT DEVELOPED JUST A FEW YEARS AGO. CUT FROM THE FLAVORFUL CHUCK SECTION NEAR THE SHOULDER BLADE, IT IS SURPRISINGLY TENDER AND TASTES MUCH MORE EXPENSIVE THAN IT IS—WHICH LIKELY ACCOUNTS FOR ITS QUICK RISE IN POPULARITY.

STEAKS
⅓ cup fresh lime juice
¼ cup extra virgin olive oil
¼ cup coarsely chopped cilantro
5 cloves garlic, minced
4 6-ounce flat-iron (boneless beef shoulder top blade) steaks

SALSA SALAD
1 seedless (English) cucumber (peeled if desired), diced
1 cup quartered grape tomatoes
½ cup diced red onion
½ cup coarsely chopped cilantro
1 poblano chile, seeded and diced (see tip)
1 jalapeño, seeded and minced (see tip)
3 tablespoons fresh lime juice
2 tablespoons extra virgin olive oil

CARAMELIZED ONIONS
2 tablespoons extra virgin olive oil
2 large sweet onions (such as Maui, Vidalia, Texas Sweet, or Walla Walla)

½ teaspoon ground chipotle chile pepper

1. For steaks, place steaks in a resealable plastic bag set in a shallow dish; set aside. In a small bowl combine lime juice, oil, cilantro, and garlic; pour over steaks in bag. Seal bag; turn to coat. Marinate in the refrigerator for 2 hours.

2. For salad, in a large bowl combine cucumber, tomatoes, onion, cilantro, poblano, and jalapeño. Toss to combine. For dressing, in a small bowl whisk together lime juice and olive oil together. Drizzle dressing over vegetables; toss to coat. Cover and refrigerate until serving time.

3. For onions, preheat oven to 400°F. Brush the inside of a Dutch oven with some of the olive oil; set aside. Cut onions in half lengthwise, remove skins, and then slice crosswise ¼ inch thick. In the Dutch oven combine the remaining olive oil, the onions, and the chipotle chile pepper. Cover and bake for 20 minutes. Uncover and let cool about 20 minutes.

4. Transfer cooled onions to a foil grilling bag or wrap onions in a double thickness of foil. Puncture the top of the foil in several places with a skewer.

5. For a charcoal grill, arrange medium-hot coals around perimeter of grill. Test for medium heat above center of grill. Place packet in center of grill rack. Cover and grill about 45 minutes or until onions are soft and amber color. (For a gas grill, preheat grill. Reduce heat to medium. Adjust for indirect cooking. Place packet over the burner that is turned off. Cover and grill as directed.)

6. Remove steaks from marinade; discard marinade. For a charcoal or gas grill, place steaks on the grill rack directly over medium-high heat. Cover and grill for 8 to 10 minutes or until an instant-read thermometer inserted horizontally into the steaks reads 135°F, turning once. Transfer steaks to a platter, cover loosely with foil and let stand for 10 minutes.

7. To serve, divide salsa salad among four serving plates. Place a steak on each plate and top with a mound of caramelized onions. Serve immediately.

Make-Ahead Directions: Salsa salad may be made and refrigerated up to 4 hours before serving.

GRILLED RIBEYES WITH HERBED ONION AND GARLIC "BUTTER"

PREP: 10 minutes COOK: 12 minutes CHILL: 30 minutes GRILL: 11 minutes MAKES: 4 servings

THE HEAT FROM JUST-OFF-THE-GRILL STEAKS MELTS THE MOUNDS OF CARAMELIZED ONIONS, GARLIC, AND HERBS SUSPENDED IN A RICH-TASTING BLEND OF COCONUT OIL AND OLIVE OIL.

2 tablespoons unrefined coconut oil
1 small onion, halved and cut into very thin slivers (about ¾ cup)
1 clove garlic, very thinly sliced
2 tablespoons extra virgin olive oil
1 tablespoon snipped fresh parsley
2 teaspoons snipped fresh thyme, rosemary, and/or oregano
4 8- to 10-ounce beef ribeye steaks, cut 1 inch thick
½ teaspoon freshly ground black pepper

1. In a medium skillet melt coconut oil over low heat. Add onion; cook for 10 to 15 minutes or until lightly browned, stirring occasionally. Add garlic; cook for 2 to 3 minutes more or until onion is golden brown, stirring occasionally.

2. Transfer onion mixture to a small bowl. Stir in olive oil, parsley, and thyme. Refrigerate, uncovered, for 30 minutes or until mixture is firm enough to mound when scooped, stirring occasionally.

3. Meanwhile, sprinkle steaks with pepper. For a charcoal or gas grill, place steaks on the grill rack directly over medium heat. Cover and grill for 11 to 15 minutes for

medium rare (145°F) or 14 to 18 minutes for medium (160°F), turning once halfway through grilling.

4. To serve, place each steak on a serving plate. Immediately scoop onion mixture evenly onto steaks.

RIBEYE SALAD WITH GRILLED BEETS

PREP: 20 minutes GRILL: 55 minutes STAND: 5 minutes MAKES: 4 servings

THE EARTHY FLAVOR OF BEETS PAIRS BEAUTIFULLY WITH THE SWEETNESS OF THE ORANGES—AND THE TOASTED PECANS ADD A BIT OF CRUNCH TO THIS MAIN-DISH SALAD THAT'S PERFECT FOR EATING OUTDOORS ON A WARM SUMMER NIGHT.

1 pound medium golden and/or red beets, scrubbed, trimmed, and cut into wedges
1 small onion, cut into thin wedges
2 sprigs fresh thyme
1 tablespoon extra virgin olive oil
Cracked black pepper
2 8-ounce boneless beef ribeye steaks, cut ¾ inch thick
2 cloves garlic, halved
2 tablespoons Mediterranean Seasoning (see recipe)
6 cups mixed greens
2 oranges, peeled, sectioned, and coarsely chopped
½ cup chopped pecans, toasted (see tip)
½ cup Bright Citrus Vinaigrette (see recipe)

1. Place beets, onion, and thyme sprigs in a foil pan. Drizzle with oil and toss to combine; sprinkle lightly with cracked black pepper. For a charcoal or gas grill, place pan on the center of the grill rack. Cover and grill 55 to 60 minutes or until tender when pierced with a knife, stirring occasionally.

2. Meanwhile, rub both sides of the steaks with cut sides of garlic; sprinkle with Mediterranean Seasoning.

3. Move beets from center of grill to make room for steaks. Add steaks to grill directly over medium heat. Cover and

grill for 11 to 15 minutes for medium rare (145°F) or 14 to 18 minutes for medium (160°F), turning once halfway through grilling. Remove foil pan and steaks from grill. Let steaks stand for 5 minutes. Discard thyme sprigs from foil pan.

4. Thinly slice steak diagonally into bite-size pieces. Divide greens among four serving plates. Top with sliced steak, beets, onion wedges, chopped oranges, and pecans. Drizzle with Bright Citrus Vinaigrette.

KOREAN-STYLE SHORT RIBS WITH SAUTÉED GINGER CABBAGE

PREP: 50 minutes COOK: 25 minutes BAKE: 10 hours CHILL: overnight MAKES: 4 servings

MAKE SURE THE LID OF YOUR DUTCH OVEN FITS VERY TIGHTLY SO THAT DURING THE VERY LONG BRAISING TIME, THE COOKING LIQUID DOESN'T ALL EVAPORATE THROUGH A GAP BETWEEN THE LID AND POT.

1 ounce dried shiitake mushrooms
1½ cups sliced scallions
1 Asian pear, peeled, cored, and chopped
1 3-inch piece fresh ginger, peeled and chopped
1 serrano chile pepper, finely chopped (seeded if desired) (see tip)
5 cloves garlic
1 tablespoon refined coconut oil
5 pounds bone-in beef short ribs
Freshly ground black pepper
4 cups Beef Bone Broth (see recipe) or no-salt-added beef broth
2 cups sliced fresh shiitake mushrooms
1 tablespoon finely shredded orange peel
⅓ cup fresh juice
Sautéed Ginger Cabbage (see recipe, below)
Finely shredded orange peel (optional)

1. Preheat oven to 325°F. Place dried shiitake mushrooms in a small bowl; add enough boiling water to cover. Let stand about 30 minutes or until rehydrated and soft. Drain, reserving the soaking liquid. Finely chop the mushrooms. Place mushrooms in a small bowl; cover and refrigerate until needed in Step 4. Set mushrooms and liquid aside.

2. For sauce, in a food processor combine scallions, Asian pear, ginger, serrano, garlic, and the reserved mushroom soaking liquid. Cover and process until smooth. Set sauce aside.

3. In a 6-quart Dutch oven heat the coconut oil over medium-high heat. Sprinkle short ribs with freshly ground black pepper. Cook ribs, in batches, in hot coconut oil about 10 minutes or until well browned on all sides, turning halfway through cooking. Return all the ribs to the pot; add sauce and Beef Bone broth. Cover the Dutch oven with a tight-fitting lid. Bake about 10 hours or until meat is very tender and falls off the bones.

4. Carefully remove the ribs from sauce. Place ribs and sauce in separate containers. Cover and refrigerate overnight. When cold, remove fat from surface of the sauce and discard. Bring the sauce to boiling over high heat; add hydrated mushrooms from Step 1 and the fresh mushrooms. Boil gently for 10 minutes to reduce sauce and intensify flavors. Return ribs to the sauce; simmer until heated through. Stir in 1 tablespoon orange peel and the orange juice. Serve with Sautéed Ginger Cabbage. If desired, sprinkle with additional orange peel.

Sautéed Ginger Cabbage: In a large skillet heat 1 tablespoon refined coconut oil over medium-high heat. Add 2 tablespoons minced fresh ginger; 2 cloves garlic, minced; and crushed red pepper to taste. Cook and stir until fragrant, about 30 seconds. Add 6 cups shredded napa, savoy, or green cabbage and 1 Asian pear, peeled, cored, and thinly sliced. Cook and stir for 3 minutes or until cabbage wilts slightly and pear softens. Stir in ½ cup unsweetened apple juice. Cover and cook about 2 minutes until cabbage is tender. Stir in ½ cup sliced scallions and 1 tablespoon sesame seeds.

BEEF SHORT RIBS WITH CITRUS-FENNEL GREMOLATA

PREP: 40 minutes GRILL: 8 minutes SLOW COOK: 9 hours (low) or 4½ hours (high) MAKES: 4 servings

GREMOLATA IS A FLAVORFUL BLEND OF PARSLEY, GARLIC, AND LEMON PEEL THAT IS SPRINKLED ON OSSO BUCCO—THE CLASSIC ITALIAN DISH OF BRAISED VEAL SHANKS—TO BRIGHTEN ITS RICH, UNCTUOUS FLAVOR. WITH THE ADDITION OF ORANGE PEEL AND FRESH FEATHERY FENNEL FRONDS, IT DOES THE SAME FOR THESE TENDER BEEF SHORT RIBS.

RIBS

2½ to 3 pounds bone-in beef short ribs

3 tablespoons Lemon-Herb Seasoning (see recipe)

1 medium fennel bulb

1 large onion, cut into large wedges

2 cups Beef Bone Broth (see recipe) or no-salt-added beef broth

2 cloves garlic, halved

PAN-ROASTED SQUASH

3 tablespoons extra virgin olive oil

1 pound butternut squash, peeled, seeded, and cut into ½-inch pieces (about 2 cups)

4 teaspoons snipped fresh thyme

Extra virgin olive oil

GREMOLATA

¼ cup snipped fresh parsley

2 tablespoons minced garlic

1½ teaspoons finely shredded lemon peel

1½ teaspoons finely shredded orange peel

1. Sprinkle short ribs with Lemon-Herb Seasoning; lightly rub into meat with your fingers; set aside. Remove fronds from fennel; set aside for Citrus-Fennel Gremolata. Trim and quarter fennel bulb.

2. For a charcoal grill, arrange medium-hot coals on one side of the grill. Test for medium heat above the side of grill without coals. Place short ribs on grill rack on side without coals; place fennel quarters and onion wedges on the rack directly over coals. Cover and grill for 8 to 10 minutes or until vegetables and ribs are just browned, turning once halfway through grilling. (For a gas grill, preheat grill, reduce heat to medium. Adjust for indirect cooking. Place ribs on grill rack over burner that is turned off; place fennel and onion on rack over burner that is turned on. Cover and grill as directed.) When cool enough to handle, coarsely chop the fennel and onion.

3. In a 5- to 6-quart slow cooker combine chopped fennel and onion, Beef Bone Broth, and garlic. Add ribs. Cover and cook on low-heat setting for 9 to 10 hours or 4½ to 5 hours on high-heat setting. Using a slotted spoon, transfer ribs to a platter; cover with foil to keep warm.

4. Meanwhile, for the squash, in a large skillet heat the 3 tablespoons oil over medium-high heat. Add squash and 3 teaspoons of the thyme, stirring to coat the squash. Arrange squash in a single layer in skillet and cook without stirring about 3 minutes or until browned on bottom sides. Turn squash pieces over; cook about 3 minutes more or until second sides are browned. Reduce heat to low; cover and cook for 10 to 15 minutes or until

tender. Sprinkle with remaining 1 teaspoon fresh thyme; drizzle with additional extra virgin olive oil.

5. For the gremolata, finely chop enough reserved fennel fronds to make ¼ cup. In a small bowl stir together the chopped fennel fronds, parsley, garlic, lemon peel, and orange peel.

6. Sprinkle gremolata over ribs. Serve with squash.

SWEDISH-STYLE BEEF PATTIES WITH MUSTARD-DILL CUCUMBER SALAD

PREP: 30 minutes COOK: 15 minutes MAKES: 4 servings

BEEF À LA LINDSTROM IS A SWEDISH HAMBURGER THAT IS TRADITIONALLY STUDDED WITH ONIONS, CAPERS, AND PICKLED BEETS SERVED WITH GRAVY AND WITHOUT A BUN. THIS ALLSPICE-INFUSED VERSION SUBSTITUTES ROASTED BEETS FOR THE SALT-LADEN PICKLED BEETS AND CAPERS AND IS TOPPED WITH A FRIED EGG.

CUCUMBER SALAD
- 2 teaspoons fresh orange juice
- 2 teaspoons white wine vinegar
- 1 teaspoon Dijon-Style Mustard (see recipe)
- 1 tablespoon extra virgin olive oil
- 1 large seedless (English) cucumber, peeled and sliced
- 2 tablespoons sliced scallions
- 1 tablespoon chopped fresh dill

BEEF PATTIES
- 1 pound ground beef
- ¼ cup finely chopped onion
- 1 tablespoon Dijon-Style Mustard (see recipe)
- ¾ teaspoon black pepper
- ½ teaspoon ground allspice
- ½ of a small beet, roasted, peeled, and finely diced*
- 2 tablespoons extra virgin olive oil
- ½ cup Beef Bone Broth (see recipe) or no-salt-added beef broth
- 4 large eggs
- 1 tablespoon finely chopped chives

1. For cucumber salad, in a large bowl whisk together orange juice, vinegar, and Dijon-Style Mustard. Slowly add olive oil in a thin stream, whisking until dressing thickens slightly. Add cucumber, scallions, and dill; toss until combined. Cover and refrigerate until serving time.

2. For beef patties, in a large bowl combine ground beef, onion, Dijon-Style Mustard, pepper, and allspice. Add roasted beet and gently mix until evenly incorporated into the meat. Shape mixture into four ½-inch-thick patties.

3. In a large skillet heat 1 tablespoon olive oil over medium-high heat. Fry patties about 8 minutes or until browned on the exterior and cooked through (160°), turning once. Transfer patties to a plate and cover loosely with foil to keep warm. Add Beef Bone Broth, stirring to scrape up browned bits from bottom of skillet. Cook about 4 minutes or until reduced by half. Drizzle patties with reduced pan juices and re-cover loosely.

4. Rinse and wipe out skillet with a paper towel. Heat the remaining 1 tablespoon olive oil over medium heat. Fry eggs in hot oil for 3 to 4 minutes or until whites are cooked but yolks remain soft and runny.

5. Place an egg on each beef patty. Sprinkle with chives and serve with cucumber salad.

*Tip: To roast beet, scrub well and place on a piece of aluminum foil. Drizzle with a little olive oil. Wrap in foil and seal tightly. Roast in a 375°F oven about 30 minutes or until a fork easily pierces beet. Let cool; slip skin off.

(Beet can be roasted up to 3 days ahead. Tightly wrap peeled roasted beets and store in the refrigerator.)

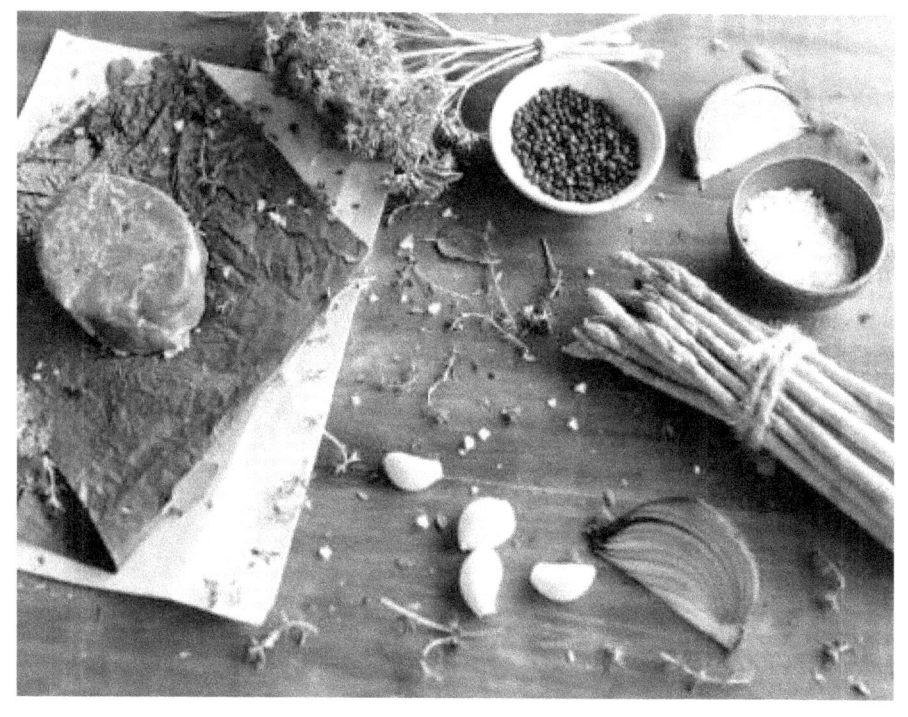

SMOTHERED BEEFBURGERS ON ARUGULA WITH ROASTED ROOT VEGETABLES

PREP: 40 minutes COOK: 35 minutes ROAST: 20 minutes MAKES: 4 servings

THERE ARE A LOT OF ELEMENTS TO THESE HEARTY BURGERS—AND THEY DO TAKE A BIT OF TIME TO PUT TOGETHER—BUT THE INCREDIBLE COMBINATION OF FLAVORS MAKES IT WELL WORTH THE EFFORT: A MEATY BURGER IS TOPPED WITH CARAMELIZED ONION AND MUSHROOM PAN SAUCE AND SERVED WITH SWEET ROASTED VEGETABLES AND PEPPERY ARUGULA.

5 tablespoons extra virgin olive oil

2 cups sliced fresh button, cremini, and/or shiitake mushrooms

3 yellow onions, thinly sliced*

2 teaspoons caraway seeds

3 carrots, peeled and cut into 1-inch chunks

2 parsnips, peeled and cut into 1-inch chunks

1 acorn squash, halved, seeded, and cut into wedges

Freshly ground black pepper

2 pounds ground beef

½ cup finely chopped onion

1 tablespoon salt-free all-purpose seasoning blend

2 cups Beef Bone Broth (see recipe) or no-salt-added beef broth

¼ cup unsweetened apple juice

1 to 2 tablespoons dry sherry or white wine vinegar

1 tablespoon Dijon-Style Mustard (see recipe)

1 tablespoon snipped fresh thyme leaves

1 tablespoon snipped fresh parsley leaves

8 cups arugula leaves

1. Preheat oven to 425°F. For sauce, in a large skillet heat 1 tablespoon of the olive oil over medium-high heat. Add mushrooms; cook and stir about 8 minutes or until well browned and tender. Using a slotted spoon, transfer the mushrooms to a plate. Return the skillet to the burner; reduce heat to medium. Add the remaining 1 tablespoon olive oil, sliced onions, and the caraway seeds. Cover and cook for 20 to 25 minutes or until onions are very soft and richly browned, stirring occasionally. (Adjust heat as needed to prevent the onions from burning.)

2. Meanwhile, for roasted root vegetables, on a large baking sheet arrange carrots, parsnips, and squash. Drizzle with 2 tablespoons olive oil and sprinkle with pepper to taste; toss to coat vegetables. Roast for 20 to 25 minutes or until tender and beginning to brown, turning once halfway through roasting. Keep vegetables warm until ready to serve.

3. For burgers, in a large bowl combine the ground beef, finely chopped onion, and seasoning blend. Divide meat mixture into four equal portions and shape into patties, about ¾ inch thick. In an extra-large skillet heat the remaining 1 tablespoon olive oil over medium-high heat. Add burgers to skillet; cook about 8 minutes or until seared on both sides, turning once. Transfer burgers to a plate.

4. Add caramelized onions, reserved mushrooms, Beef Bone Broth, apple juice, sherry, and Dijon-Style Mustard to the skillet, stirring to combine. Return burgers to skillet. Bring to simmering. Cook until burgers are done (160°F), about

7 to 8 minutes. Stir in fresh thyme, parsley, and pepper to taste.

5. To serve, arrange 2 cups of arugula on each of four serving plates. Divide the roasted vegetables among the salads, then top with burgers. Generously spoon the onion mixture on the burgers.

*Tip: A mandoline slicer is a great help in thinly slicing onions.

GRILLED BEEFBURGERS WITH SESAME-CRUSTED TOMATOES

PREP: 30 minutes STAND: 20 minutes GRILL: 10 minutes MAKES: 4 servings

CRISP, GOLDEN-BROWN SESAME-CRUSTED SLICES OF TOMATO STAND IN FOR THE TRADITIONAL SESAME SEED BUN IN THESE SMOKY BURGERS. SERVE THEM WITH A KNIFE AND FORK.

- 4 ½-inch-thick red or green tomato slices*
- 1¼ pounds lean ground beef
- 1 tablespoon Smoky Seasoning (see recipe)
- 1 large egg
- ¾ cup almond meal
- ¼ cup sesame seeds
- ¼ teaspoon black pepper
- 1 small red onion, halved and sliced
- 1 tablespoon extra virgin olive oil
- ¼ cup refined coconut oil
- 1 small head Bibb lettuce
- Paleo Ketchup (see recipe)
- Dijon-Style Mustard (see recipe)

1. Place tomato slices on a double layer of paper towels. Top tomatoes with another double layer of paper towels. Press down lightly on paper towels so they stick to the tomatoes. Let stand at room temperature for 20 to 30 minutes so some of the tomato juice is absorbed.

2. Meanwhile, in a large bowl combine ground beef and Smoky Seasoning. Shape into four ½-inch-thick patties.

3. In a shallow bowl lightly beat egg with a fork. In another shallow bowl combine almond meal, sesame seeds, and

pepper. Dip each tomato slice into the egg, turning to coat. Allow excess egg to drip off. Dip each tomato slice into almond meal mixture, turning to coat. Place coated tomatoes on a flat plate; set aside. Toss onion slices with olive oil; place onion slices in a grill basket.

4. For a charcoal or gas grill, place onions in basket and beef patties on grill rack over medium heat. Cover and grill for 10 to 12 minutes or onions are golden brown and lightly charred and patties are done (160°), stirring onions occasionally and turning patties once.

5. Meanwhile, in a large skillet heat oil over medium heat. Add tomato slices; cook for 8 to 10 minutes or until golden brown, turning once. (If tomatoes brown too quickly, reduce heat to medium-low. If necessary, add additional oil.) Drain on a paper towel-lined plate.

6. To serve, divide lettuce among four serving plates. Top with patties, onions, Paleo Ketchup, Dijon-Style Mustard, and sesame-crusted tomatoes.

*Note: You'll probably need 2 large tomatoes. If using red tomatoes, choose tomatoes that are just ripe but still slightly firm.

BURGERS ON A STICK WITH BABA GHANOUSH DIPPING SAUCE

SOAK: 15 minutes PREP: 20 minutes GRILL: 35 minutes MAKES: 4 servings

BABA GHANOUSH IS A MIDDLE EASTERN SPREAD MADE FROM SMOKY GRILLED EGGPLANT PUREED WITH OLIVE OIL, LEMON, GARLIC, AND TAHINI, A PASTE MADE FROM GROUND SESAME SEEDS. A SPRINKLING OF SESAME SEEDS IS FINE, BUT WHEN THEY ARE MADE INTO OIL OR PASTE, THEY BECOME A CONCENTRATED SOURCE OF LINOLEIC ACID, WHICH CAN CONTRIBUTE TO INFLAMMATION. THE PINE NUT BUTTER USED HERE MAKES A FINE SUBSTITUTE.

- 4 dried tomatoes
- 1½ pounds lean ground beef
- 3 to 4 tablespoons finely chopped onion
- 1 tablespoon finely snipped fresh oregano and/or finely snipped fresh mint or ½ teaspoon dried oregano, crushed
- ¼ teaspoon cayenne pepper
- Baba Ghanoush Dipping Sauce (see recipe, below)

1. Soak eight 10-inch wooden skewers in water for 30 minutes. Meanwhile, in a small bowl pour boiling water over tomatoes; let stand for 5 minutes to rehydrate. Drain tomatoes and pat dry with paper towels.

2. In large bowl combine chopped tomatoes, ground beef, onion, oregano, and cayenne pepper. Divide meat mixture into eight portions; roll each portion into a ball. Remove skewers from water; pat dry. Thread one ball onto a skewer and shape into a long oval around the skewer, starting just below the pointed tip and leaving enough

room on the other end to be able to hold the stick. Repeat with remaining skewers and balls.

3. For a charcoal or gas grill, place beef skewers on a grill rack directly over medium heat. Cover and grill about 6 minutes or until done (160°F), turning once halfway through grilling. Serve with Baba Ghanoush Dipping Sauce.

Baba Ghanoush Dipping Sauce: Poke 2 medium eggplants in several places with a fork. For a charcoal or gas grill, place eggplants on a grill rack directly over medium heat. Cover and grill for 10 minutes or until charred on all sides, turning several times during grilling. Remove eggplants and carefully wrap in foil. Place wrapped eggplants back on the grill rack but not directly over the coals. Cover and grill for 25 to 35 minutes more or until collapsed and very tender. Cool. Halve eggplants and scrape out the flesh; place flesh in a food processor. Add ¼ cup Pine Nut Butter (see recipe); ¼ cup fresh lemon juice; 2 cloves garlic, minced; 1 tablespoon extra virgin olive oil; 2 to 3 tablespoons snipped fresh parsley; and ½ teaspoon ground cumin. Cover and process just until almost smooth. If sauce is too thick for dipping, stir in enough water to make desired consistency.

SMOKY STUFFED SWEET PEPPERS

PREP: 20 minutes COOK: 8 minutes BAKE: 30 minutes MAKES: 4 servings

MAKE THIS FAMILY FAVORITE WITH A MIX OF COLORED SWEET PEPPERS FOR AN EYE-CATCHING DISH. THE FIRE-ROASTED TOMATOES ARE A FINE EXAMPLE OF HOW TO ADD GREAT TASTE TO FOOD IN A HEALTHY WAY. THE SIMPLE ACT OF SLIGHTLY CHARRING THE TOMATOES BEFORE THEY ARE CANNED (WITHOUT SALT) BUMPS UP THEIR FLAVOR.

- 4 large green, red, yellow, and/or orange sweet peppers
- 1 pound ground beef
- 1 tablespoon Smoky Seasoning (see recipe)
- 1 tablespoon extra virgin olive oil
- 1 small yellow onion, chopped
- 3 cloves garlic, minced
- 1 small head cauliflower, cored and broken into florets
- 1 15-ounce can no-salt-added diced fire-roasted tomatoes, drained
- ¼ cup finely chopped fresh parsley
- ½ teaspoon black pepper
- ⅛ teaspoon cayenne pepper
- ½ cup Walnut Crumb Topping (see recipe, below)

1. Preheat oven to 375°F. Cut sweet peppers in half vertically. Remove stems, seeds, and membranes; discard. Set pepper halves aside.

2. Place ground beef in a medium bowl; sprinkle with Smoky Seasoning. Use your hands to gently mix seasoning into meat.

3. In a large skillet heat olive oil over medium heat. Add meat, onion, and garlic; cook until meat is browned and onion is

tender, stirring with a wooden spoon to break up meat. Remove skillet from heat.

4. In a food processor process cauliflower florets until very finely chopped. (If you don't have a food processor, grate the cauliflower on a box grater.) Measure 3 cups of the cauliflower. Add to ground beef mixture in skillet. (If there is any remaining cauliflower, save it for another use.) Stir in drained tomatoes, parsley, black pepper, and cayenne pepper.

5. Fill pepper halves with ground beef mixture, packing it lightly and mounding slightly. Arrange filled pepper halves in a baking dish. Bake for 30 to 35 minutes or until peppers are crisp-tender.* Top with Walnut Crumb Topping. If desired, return to oven for 5 minutes to crisp topping before serving.

Walnut Crumb Topping: In a medium skillet heat 1 tablespoon extra virgin olive oil over medium low heat. Stir in 1 teaspoon dried thyme, 1 teaspoon smoked paprika, and ¼ teaspoon garlic powder. Add 1 cup very finely chopped walnuts. Cook and stir about 5 minutes or until walnuts are golden brown and lightly toasted. Stir in a dash or two of cayenne pepper. Let cool completely. Store leftover topping in a tightly sealed container in the refrigerator until ready to use. Makes 1 cup.

*Note: If using green peppers, bake for an additional 10 minutes.

BISON BURGERS WITH CABERNET ONIONS AND ARUGULA

PREP: 30 minutes COOK: 18 minutes GRILL: 10 minutes MAKES: 4 servings

BISON HAS A VERY LOW FAT CONTENT AND WILL COOK 30% TO 50% FASTER THAN BEEF. THE MEAT RETAINS ITS RED COLOR AFTER COOKING, SO COLOR IS NOT AN INDICATOR OF DONENESS. BECAUSE BISON IS SO LEAN, DO NOT COOK IT BEYOND AN INTERNAL TEMPERATURE OF 155°F.

- 2 tablespoons extra virgin olive oil
- 2 large sweet onions, thinly sliced
- ¾ cup Cabernet Sauvignon or other dry red wine
- 1 teaspoon Mediterranean Seasoning (see recipe)
- ¼ cup extra virgin olive oil
- ¼ cup balsamic vinegar
- 1 tablespoon finely chopped shallot
- 1 tablespoon snipped fresh basil
- 1 small clove garlic, minced
- 1 pound ground bison
- ¼ cup Basil Pesto (see recipe)
- 5 cups arugula
- Raw unsalted pistachios, toasted (see tip)

1. In a large skillet heat the 2 tablespoons oil over medium-low heat. Add onions. Cook, covered, for 10 to 15 minutes or until onions are tender, stirring occasionally. Uncover; cook and stir over medium-high heat for 3 to 5 minutes or until onions are golden. Add wine; cook about 5 minutes or until most of the wine evaporates. Sprinkle with Mediterranean Seasoning; keep warm.

2. Meanwhile, for vinaigrette, in a screw-top jar combine the ¼ cup olive oil, vinegar, shallot, basil, and garlic. Cover and shake well.

3. In a large bowl lightly mix ground bison and Basil Pesto. Lightly shape meat mixture into four ¾-inch-thick patties.

4. For a charcoal or gas grill, place patties on a lightly greased grill rack directly over medium heat. Cover and grill about 10 minutes to desired doneness (145°F for medium rare or 155°F for medium), turning once halfway through grilling.

5. Place arugula in a large bowl. Drizzle vinaigrette over arugula; toss to coat. To serve, divide onions among four serving plates; top each with a bison burger. Top burgers with arugula and sprinkle with pistachios.

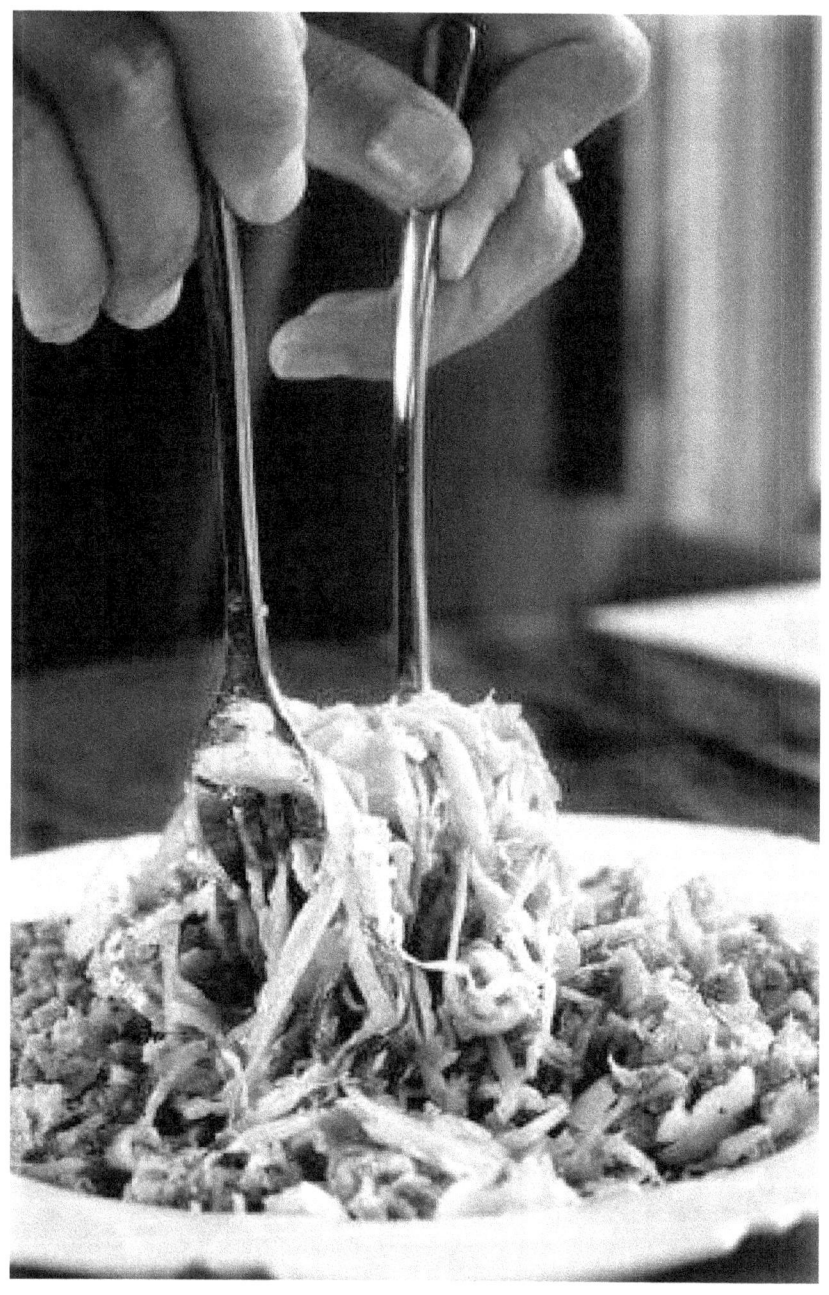

BISON AND LAMB MEAT LOAF ON CHARD AND SWEET POTATOES

PREP: 1 hour COOK: 20 minutes BAKE: 1 hour STAND: 10 minutes MAKES: 4 servings

THIS IS OLD-FASHIONED COMFORT FOOD WITH A MODERN TWIST. A RED-WINE PAN SAUCE GIVES THE MEAT LOAF A FLAVOR BOOST, AND THE GARLICKY CHARD AND SWEET POTATOES MASHED WITH CASHEW CREAM AND COCONUT OIL OFFER INCREDIBLE NUTRITIONAL CONTENT.

2 tablespoons olive oil
1 cup finely chopped cremini mushrooms
½ cup finely chopped red onion (1 medium)
½ cup finely chopped celery (1 stalk)
⅓ cup finely chopped carrot (1 small)
½ of a small apple, cored, peeled, and shredded
2 cloves garlic, minced
½ teaspoon Mediterranean Seasoning (see recipe)
1 large egg, lightly beaten
1 tablespoon snipped fresh sage
1 tablespoon snipped fresh thyme
8 ounces ground bison
8 ounces ground lamb or beef
¾ cup dry red wine
1 medium shallot, finely chopped
¾ cup Beef Bone Broth (see recipe) or no-salt-added beef broth
Mashed Sweet Potatoes (see recipe, below)
Garlicky Swiss Chard (see recipe, below)

1. Preheat oven to 350°F. In a large skillet heat oil over medium heat. Add mushrooms, onion, celery, and carrot; cook and stir about 5 minutes or until vegetables are

softened. Reduce heat to low; add shredded apple and garlic. Cook, covered, about 5 minutes or until vegetables are very tender. Remove from heat; stir in Mediterranean Seasoning.

2. Using a slotted spoon, transfer mushroom mixture to a large bowl, reserving drippings in skillet. Stir in egg, sage, and thyme. Add ground bison and ground lamb; lightly mix. Spoon meat mixture into a 2-quart rectangular baking dish; shape into a 7×4-inch rectangle. Bake about 1 hour or until an instant-read thermometer registers 155°F. Let stand for 10 minutes. Carefully remove meat loaf to a serving platter. Cover and keep warm.

3. For the pan sauce, scrape drippings and crusty browned bits from the baking dish into reserved drippings in the skillet. Add wine and shallot. Bring to boiling over medium heat; cook until reduced by half. Add Beef Bone Broth; cook and stir until reduced by half. Remove skillet from heat.

4. To serve, divide Mashed Sweet Potatoes among four serving plates; top with some of the Garlicky Swiss Chard. Slice meat loaf; place slices on Garlicky Swiss Chard and drizzle with the pan sauce.

Mashed Sweet Potatoes: Peel and coarsely chop 4 medium sweet potatoes. In a large saucepan cook potatoes in enough boiling water to cover for 15 minutes or until tender; drain. Mash with a potato masher. Add ½ cup Cashew Cream (see recipe) and 2 tablespoons unrefined coconut oil; mash until smooth. Keep warm.

Garlicky Swiss Chard: Remove stems from 2 bunches Swiss chard and discard. Coarsely chop leaves. In a large skillet heat 2 tablespoons olive oil over medium heat. Add Swiss chard and 2 cloves garlic, minced; cook until chard is wilted, tossing occasionally with tongs.

APPLE-CURRANT-SAUCED BISON MEATBALLS WITH ZUCCHINI PAPPARDELLE

PREP: 25 minutes BAKE: 15 minutes COOK: 18 minutes MAKES: 4 servings

THE MEATBALLS WILL BE VERY WET AS YOU FORM THEM. TO KEEP THE MEAT MIXTURE FROM STICKING TO YOUR HANDS, KEEP A BOWL OF COOL WATER HANDY AND WET YOUR HANDS OCCASIONALLY AS YOU WORK. CHANGE THE WATER A COUPLE OF TIMES AS YOU MAKE THE MEATBALLS.

MEATBALLS
- Olive oil
- ½ cup coarsely chopped red onion
- 2 cloves garlic, minced
- 1 egg, lightly beaten
- ½ cup finely chopped button mushrooms and stems
- 2 tablespoon snipped fresh Italian (flat-leaf) parsley
- 2 teaspoons olive oil
- 1 pound ground bison (coarse ground if available)

APPLE-CURRANT SAUCE
- 2 tablespoons olive oil
- 2 large Granny Smith apples, peeled, cored, and finely chopped
- 2 shallots, minced
- 2 tablespoons fresh lemon juice
- ½ cup Chicken Bone Broth (see recipe) or no-salt-added chicken broth
- 2 to 3 tablespoons dried currants

ZUCCHINI PAPPARDELLE
- 6 zucchini
- 2 tablespoons olive oil

¼ cup finely chopped scallions

½ teaspoon crushed red pepper

2 cloves garlic, minced

1. For meatballs, preheat oven to 375°F. Lightly brush a rimmed baking sheet with olive oil; set aside. In a food processor or blender combine onion and garlic. Pulse until smooth. Transfer onion mixture to a medium bowl. Add egg, mushrooms, parsley, and 2 teaspoons oil; stir to combine. Add ground bison; mix lightly but well. Divide meat mixture into 16 portions; shape into meatballs. Place meatballs, evenly spaced, on the prepared baking sheet. Bake for 15 minutes; set aside.

2. For sauce, in a skillet heat 2 tablespoons oil over medium heat. Add apples and shallots; cook and stir for 6 to 8 minutes or until very tender. Stir in lemon juice. Transfer mixture to a food processor or blender. Cover and process or blend until smooth; return to the skillet. Stir in Chicken Bone Broth and currants. Bring to boiling; reduce heat. Simmer, uncovered, for 8 to 10 minutes, stirring frequently. Add meatballs; cook and stir over low heat until heated through.

3. Meanwhile, for pappardelle, trim ends of zucchini. Using a mandoline or very sharp vegetable peeler, shave zucchini into thin ribbons. (To keep the ribbons intact, stop shaving once you reach the seeds in the center of the squash.) In a extra-large skillet heat 2 tablespoons oil over medium heat. Stir in scallions, crushed red pepper, and garlic; cook and stir for 30 seconds. Add zucchini ribbons. Cook and gently stir about 3 minutes or just until wilted.

4. To serve, divide pappardelle among four serving plates; top with meatballs and apple-currant sauce.

BISON-PORCINI BOLOGNESE WITH ROASTED GARLIC SPAGHETTI SQUASH

PREP: 30 minutes COOK: 1 hour 30 minutes BAKE: 35 minutes MAKES: 6 servings

IF YOU THOUGHT YOU'D EATEN YOUR LAST DISH OF SPAGHETTI WITH MEAT SAUCE WHEN YOU ADOPTED THE PALEO DIET®, THINK AGAIN. THIS RICH BOLOGNESE FLAVORED WITH GARLIC, RED WINE, AND EARTHY PORCINI MUSHROOMS IS LADELED OVER SWEET, TOOTHSOME STRANDS OF SPAGHETTI SQUASH. YOU WON'T MISS THE PASTA ONE BIT.

1 ounce dried porcini mushrooms

1 cup boiling water

3 tablespoons extra virgin olive oil

1 pound ground bison

1 cup finely chopped carrots (2)

½ cup chopped onion (1 medium)

½ cup finely chopped celery (1 stalk)

4 cloves garlic, minced

3 tablespoons salt-free tomato paste

½ cup red wine

2 15-ounce cans no-salt-added crushed tomatoes

1 teaspoon dried oregano, crushed

1 teaspoon dried thyme, crushed

½ teaspoon black pepper

1 medium spaghetti squash (2½ to 3 pounds)

1 bulb garlic

1. In a small bowl combine the porcini mushrooms and boiling water; let stand for 15 minutes. Strain through a sieve lined with 100%-cotton cheesecloth, reserving the soaking liquid. Chop the mushrooms; set side.

2. In a 4- to 5-quart Dutch oven heat 1 tablespoon of the olive oil over medium heat. Add ground bison, carrots, onion, celery, and garlic. Cook until meat is browned and vegetables are tender, stirring with a wooden spoon to break up meat. Add tomato paste; cook and stir for 1 minute. Add red wine; cook and stir for 1 minute. Stir in porcini mushrooms, tomatoes, oregano, thyme, and pepper. Add reserved mushroom liquid, being careful to avoid adding any sand or grit that may be present in the bottom of the bowl. Bring to boiling, stirring occasionally; reduce heat to low. Simmer, covered, for 1½ to 2 hours or until desired consistency.

3. Meanwhile, preheat oven to 375°F. Halve squash lengthwise; scrape out seeds. Place squash halves, cut sides down, in a large baking dish. Using a fork, prick the skin all over. Cut off the top ½ inch of the head of garlic. Place the garlic, cut end up, in the baking dish with the squash. Drizzle with the remaining 1 tablespoon olive oil. Bake for 35 to 45 minutes or until squash and garlic are tender.

4. Using a spoon and fork, remove and shred the squash flesh from each squash half; transfer to a bowl and cover to keep warm. When the garlic is cool enough to handle, squeeze the bulb from the bottom to pop out the cloves. Use a fork to mash the garlic cloves. Stir mashed garlic into the squash, distributing garlic evenly. To serve, spoon sauce over squash mixture.

BISON CHILI CON CARNE

PREP: 25 minutes COOK: 1 hour 10 minutes MAKES: 4 servings

UNSWEETENED CHOCOLATE, COFFEE, AND CINNAMON ADD INTEREST TO THIS HEARTY FAVORITE. IF YOU'D LIKE EVEN MORE SMOKY FLAVOR, SUBSTITUTE 1 TABLESPOON OF SWEET SMOKED PAPRIKA FOR THE REGULAR PAPRIKA.

3 tablespoons extra virgin olive oil

1 pound ground bison

½ cup chopped onion (1 medium)

2 cloves garlic, minced

2 14.5-ounce cans diced no-salt-added tomatoes, undrained

1 6-ounce can salt-free tomato paste

1 cup Beef Bone Broth (see recipe) or no-salt-added beef broth

½ cup strong coffee

2 ounces 99% cacao baking bar, chopped

1 tablespoon paprika

1 teaspoon ground cumin

1 teaspoon dried oregano

1½ teaspoons Smoky Seasoning (see recipe)

½ teaspoon ground cinnamon

⅓ cup pepitas

1 teaspoon olive oil

½ cup Cashew Cream (see recipe)

1 teaspoon fresh lime juice

½ cup fresh cilantro leaves

4 lime wedges

1. In a Dutch oven heat the 3 tablespoons olive oil over medium heat. Add ground bison, onion, and garlic; cook about 5 minutes or until meat is browned, stirring with a wooden spoon to break up meat. Stir in undrained

tomatoes, tomato paste, Beef Bone Broth, coffee, baking chocolate, paprika, cumin, oregano, 1 teaspoon of the Smoky Seasoning, and cinnamon. Bring to boiling; reduce heat. Simmer, covered, for 1 hour, stirring occasionally.

2. Meanwhile, in a small skillet toast pepitas in the 1 teaspoon olive oil over medium heat until they start to pop and turn golden. Place pepitas in a small bowl; add the remaining ½ teaspoon Smoky Seasoning; toss to coat.

3. In a small bowl combine Cashew Cream and lime juice.

4. To serve, ladle chili into bowls. Top servings with Cashew Cream, pepitas, and cilantro. Serve with lime wedges.

MOROCCAN-SPICED BISON STEAKS WITH GRILLED LEMONS

PREP: 10 minutes GRILL: 10 minutes MAKES: 4 servings

SERVE THESE QUICK-TO-FIX STEAKS WITH COOL AND CRISP SPICED CARROT SLAW (SEE RECIPE). IF YOU'RE CRAVING A TREAT, GRILLED PINEAPPLE WITH COCONUT CREAM (SEE RECIPE) WOULD BE A GREAT WAY TO END THE MEAL.

2 tablespoons ground cinnamon

2 tablespoons paprika

1 tablespoon garlic powder

¼ teaspoon cayenne pepper

4 6-ounce bison filet mignon steaks, cut ¾ to 1 inch thick

2 lemons, halved horizontally

1. In a small bowl stir together the cinnamon, paprika, garlic powder, and cayenne pepper. Pat steaks dry with paper towels. Rub both sides of steaks with the spice mixture.

2. For a charcoal or gas grill, place steaks on the grill rack directly over medium heat. Cover and grill for 10 to 12 minutes for medium rare (145°F) or 12 to 15 minutes for medium (155°F), turning once halfway through grilling. Meanwhile, place lemon halves, cut sides down, on grill rack. Grill for 2 to 3 minutes or until slightly charred and juicy.

3. Serve with grilled lemon halves to squeeze over steaks.

HERBES DE PROVENCE-RUBBED BISON SIRLOIN ROAST

PREP: 15 minutes COOK: 15 minutes ROAST: 1 hour 15 minutes STAND: 15 minutes MAKES: 4 servings

HERBES DE PROVENCE IS A BLEND OF DRIED HERBS THAT GROW IN PROFUSION IN THE SOUTH OF FRANCE. THE MIX USUALLY CONTAINS SOME COMBINATION OF BASIL, FENNEL SEEDS, LAVENDER, MARJORAM, ROSEMARY, SAGE, SUMMER SAVORY, AND THYME. IT FLAVORS THIS VERY AMERICAN ROAST BEAUTIFULLY.

1 3-pound bison sirloin roast
3 tablespoons herbes de Provence
4 tablespoons extra virgin olive oil
3 cloves garlic, minced
4 small parsnips, peeled and chopped
2 ripe pears, cored and chopped
½ cup unsweetened pear nectar
1 to 2 teaspoons fresh thyme

1. Preheat oven to 375°F. Trim fat from roast. In a small bowl combine Herbes de Provence, 2 tablespoons of the olive oil, and garlic; rub over the entire roast.

2. Place the roast on a rack in a shallow roasting pan. Insert an oven-going thermometer into the center of the roast.* Roast, uncovered, for 15 minutes. Reduce oven temperature to 300°F. Roast for 60 to 65 minutes more or until meat thermometer registers 140°F (medium rare). Cover with foil and let stand for 15 minutes.

3. Meanwhile, in a large skillet heat the remaining 2 tablespoons olive oil over medium heat. Add parsnips and pears; cook for 10 minutes or until parsnips are crisp-tender, stirring occasionally. Add pear nectar; cook about 5 minutes or until sauce is slightly thickened. Sprinkle with thyme.

4. Thinly slice roast across the grain. Serve meat with parsnips and pears.

*Tip: Bison is very lean and cooks faster than beef. Additionally, the color of the meat is redder than beef, so you can't rely on a visual cue to determine doneness. You will need a meat thermometer to let you know when the meat is done. An oven-going thermometer is ideal, though not a necessity.

COFFEE-BRAISED BISON SHORT RIBS WITH TANGERINE GREMOLATA AND CELERY ROOT MASH

PREP: 15 minutes COOK: 2 hours 45 minutes MAKES: 6 servings

BISON SHORT RIBS ARE BIG AND MEATY. THEY REQUIRE A GOOD LONG COOK IN LIQUID TO GET TENDER. GREMOLATA MADE WITH TANGERINE PEEL BRIGHTENS UP THE FLAVOR OF THIS HEARTY DISH.

MARINADE
- 2 cups water
- 3 cups strong coffee, chilled
- 2 cups fresh tangerine juice
- 2 tablespoons snipped fresh rosemary
- 1 teaspoon coarsely ground black pepper
- 4 pounds bison short ribs, cut between ribs to separate

BRAISE
- 2 tablespoons olive oil
- 1 teaspoon black pepper
- 2 cups chopped onions
- ½ cup chopped shallots
- 6 garlic cloves, chopped
- 1 jalapeño chile, seeded and chopped (see tip)
- 1 cup strong coffee
- 1 cup Beef Bone Broth (see recipe) or no-salt-added beef broth
- ¼ cup Paleo Ketchup (see recipe)
- 2 tablespoons Dijon-Style Mustard (see recipe)
- 3 tablespoons cider vinegar
- Celery Root Mash (see recipe, below)
- Tangerine Gremolata (see recipe, right)

1. For the marinade, in a large nonreactive container (glass or stainless steel) combine water, chilled coffee, tangerine juice, rosemary, and black pepper. Add ribs. Place a plate on top of ribs if necessary to keep them submerged. Cover and chill 4 to 6 hours, rearranging and stirring once.

2. For the braise, preheat oven to 325°F. Drain ribs, discarding marinade. Pat ribs dry with paper towels. In a large Dutch oven heat olive oil over medium-high heat. Season ribs with black pepper. Brown ribs in batches until browned on all sides, about 5 minutes per batch. Transfer to a large plate.

3. Add onions, shallots, garlic, and jalapeño to pot. Reduce heat to medium, cover, and cook until vegetables are soft, stirring occasionally, about 10 minutes. Add coffee and broth; stir, scraping up browned bits. Add Paleo Ketchup, Dijon-Style Mustard, and vinegar. Bring to boiling. Add ribs. Cover and transfer to oven. Cook until meat is tender, about 2 hours 15 minutes, stirring gently and rearranging ribs once or twice.

4. Transfer ribs to a plate; tent with foil to keep warm. Spoon fat from surface of sauce. Boil sauce until reduced to 2 cups, about 5 minutes. Divide Celery Root Mash among 6 plates; top with ribs and sauce. Sprinkle with Tangerine Gremolata.

Celery Root Mash: In a large saucepan combine 3 pounds celery root, peeled and cut into 1-inch pieces and 4 cups Chicken Bone Broth (see recipe) or unsalted chicken broth. Bring to boiling; reduce heat. Drain celery root, reserving broth. Return celery root to saucepan. Add 1 tablespoon olive oil and 2 teaspoons snipped fresh thyme. Using a potato masher, mash the celery root, adding reserved broth, a few tablespoons at a time, as needed to achieve desired consistency.

Tangerine Gremolata: In a small bowl combine ½ cup snipped fresh parsley, 2 tablespoons finely shredded tangerine peel, and 2 cloves minced garlic.

BEEF BONE BROTH

PREP: 25 minutes ROAST: 1 hour COOK: 8 hours MAKES: 8 to 10 cups

BONY OXTAILS MAKE AN EXTREMELY RICH-TASTING BROTH THAT CAN BE USED IN ANY RECIPE THAT CALLS FOR BEEF BROTH—OR SIMPLY ENJOYED AS A PICK-ME-UP IN A MUG ANY TIME OF DAY. THOUGH THEY ACTUALLY USED TO COME FROM AN OX, OXTAILS NOW COME FROM A BEEF ANIMAL.

5 carrots, roughly chopped

5 stalks celery, roughly chopped

2 yellow onions, unpeeled, halved

8 ounces white mushrooms

1 bulb garlic, unpeeled, halved

2 pounds oxtail bones or beef bones

2 tomatoes

12 cups cold water

3 bay leaves

1. Preheat oven to 400°F. In a large rimmed baking sheet or shallow baking pan arrange the carrots, celery, onions, mushrooms, and garlic; place the bones on top of the vegetables. In a food processor pulse tomatoes until smooth. Spread tomatoes over the bones to coat (it's okay if some of the puree drips onto the pan and the vegetables). Roast for 1 to 1½ hours or until bones are deep brown and the vegetables are caramelized. Transfer bones and vegetables to a 10- to 12-quart Dutch oven or stockpot. (If some of the tomato mixture caramelizes on the bottom of the pan, add 1 cup of hot water to the pan and scrape up any bits. Pour the liquid over the bones and

vegetables and reduce water amount by 1 cup.) Add the cold water and bay leaves.

2. Slowly bring the mixture to a simmer over medium-high to high heat. Reduce heat; cover and simmer broth for 8 to 10 hours, stirring occasionally.

3. Strain broth; discard bones and vegetables. Cool broth; transfer broth to storage containers and refrigerate for up to 5 days; freeze for up to 3 months.*

Slow Cooker Directions: For a 6- to 8-quart slow cooker, use 1 pound beef bones, 3 carrots, 3 stalks celery, 1 yellow onion, and 1 bulb garlic. Puree 1 tomato and rub onto the bones. Roast as directed, then transfer the bones and vegetables to the slow cooker. Scrape off any caramelized tomato as directed and add to the slow cooker. Add enough water to cover. Cover and cook on high-heat setting until broth comes to boiling, about 4 hours. Reduce to low-heat setting; cook for 12 to 24 hours. Strain broth; discard bones and vegetables. Store as directed.

*Tip: To easily skim fat off broth, store broth in a covered container in the refrigerator overnight. Fat will rise to the top and form a firm layer that can easily be scraped off. Broth may thicken after chilling.

TUNISIAN SPICE-RUBBED PORK SHOULDER WITH SPICY SWEET POTATO FRIES

PREP: 25 minutes ROAST: 4 hours BAKE: 30 minutes MAKES: 4 servings

THIS IS A GREAT DISH TO MAKE ON A COOL FALL DAY. THE MEAT ROASTS FOR HOURS IN THE OVEN, MAKING YOUR HOUSE SMELL WONDERFUL AND GIVING YOU TIME TO DO OTHER THINGS. OVEN-BAKED SWEET POTATO FRIES DON'T GET CRISP IN THE SAME WAY THAT WHITE POTATOES DO, BUT THEY ARE DELICIOUS IN THEIR OWN WAY, ESPECIALLY WHEN DIPPED IN GARLICKY MAYONNAISE.

PORK

- 1 2½- to 3-pound bone-in pork shoulder roast
- 2 teaspoons ground ancho chile pepper
- 2 teaspoons ground cumin
- 1 teaspoon caraway seeds, lightly crushed
- 1 teaspoon ground coriander
- ½ teaspoon ground turmeric
- ¼ teaspoon ground cinnamon
- 3 tablespoons olive oil

FRIES

- 4 medium sweet potatoes (about 2 pounds), peeled and cut into ½-inch-thick wedges
- ½ teaspoon crushed red pepper
- ½ teaspoon onion powder
- ½ teaspoon garlic powder
- Olive oil
- 1 onion, thinly sliced
- Paleo Aïoli (Garlic Mayo) (see recipe)

1. Preheat oven to 300°F. Trim fat from meat. In a small bowl combine ground ancho chile pepper, ground cumin, caraway seeds, coriander, turmeric, and cinnamon. Sprinkle meat with spice mixture; using your fingers, rub evenly into meat.

2. In an ovenproof 5- to 6-quart Dutch oven heat 1 tablespoon of the olive oil over medium-high heat. Brown pork on all sides in hot oil. Cover and roast about 4 hours or until very tender and meat thermometer registers 190°F. Remove Dutch oven from oven. Let stand, covered, while you prepare the sweet potato fries and the onions, reserving 1 tablespoon of the fat in the Dutch oven.

3. Increase oven temperature to 400°F. For the sweet potato fries, in a large bowl combine sweet potatoes, the remaining 2 tablespoons olive oil, crushed red pepper, onion powder, and garlic powder; toss to coat. Line one large or two small baking sheets with foil; brush with additional olive oil. Arrange sweet potatoes in a single layer on the prepared baking sheet(s). Bake about 30 minutes or until tender, turning the sweet potatoes once halfway through baking.

4. Meanwhile, remove meat from Dutch oven; cover with foil to keep warm. Drain drippings, reserving 1 tablespoon fat. Return the reserved fat to Dutch oven. Add onion; cook over medium heat about 5 minutes or until just softened, stirring occasionally.

5. Transfer the pork and onion to a serving platter. Using two forks, pull the pork into large shreds. Serve pork and fries with Paleo Aïoli.

CUBAN GRILLED PORK SHOULDER

PREP: 15 minutes MARINATE: 24 hours GRILL: 2 hours 30 minutes STAND: 10 minutes
MAKES: 6 to 8 servings

KNOWN AS "LECHON ASADO" IN ITS COUNTRY OF ORIGIN, THIS PORK ROAST IS MARINATED IN A COMBINATION OF FRESH CITRUS JUICES, SPICES, CRUSHED RED PEPPER, AND AN ENTIRE BULB OF MINCED GARLIC. COOKING IT OVER HOT COALS AFTER AN OVERNIGHT SOAK IN THE MARINADE INFUSES IT WITH AMAZING FLAVOR.

1 bulb garlic, cloves separated, peeled, and minced
1 cup coarsely chopped onions
1 cup olive oil
1⅓ cups fresh lime juice
⅔ cup fresh orange juice
1 tablespoon ground cumin
1 tablespoon dried oregano, crushed
2 teaspoons freshly ground black pepper
1 teaspoon crushed red pepper
1 4- to 5-pound boneless pork shoulder roast

1. For marinade, separate garlic head into cloves. Peel and mince cloves; place in a large bowl. Add onions, olive oil, lime juice, orange juice, cumin, oregano, black pepper, and crushed red pepper. Stir well and set aside.

2. Using a boning knife, deeply puncture pork roast all over. Carefully lower roast into the marinade, submerging it as much as possible in the liquid. Cover bowl tightly with plastic wrap. Marinate in the refrigerator for 24 hours, turning once.

3. Remove pork from marinade. Pour marinade into a medium saucepan. Bring to boiling; boil for 5 minutes. Remove from heat and let cool. Set aside.

4. For a charcoal grill, arrange medium-hot coals around a drip pan. Test for medium heat above the pan. Place meat on grill rack over drip pan. Cover and grill for 2½ to 3 hours or until an instant-read thermometer inserted into center of roast registers 140°F. (For a gas grill, preheat grill. Reduce heat to medium. Adjust for indirect cooking. Place meat on grill rack over burner that is turned off. Cover and grill as directed.) Remove meat from grill. Cover loosely with foil and let stand for 10 minutes before carving or pulling.

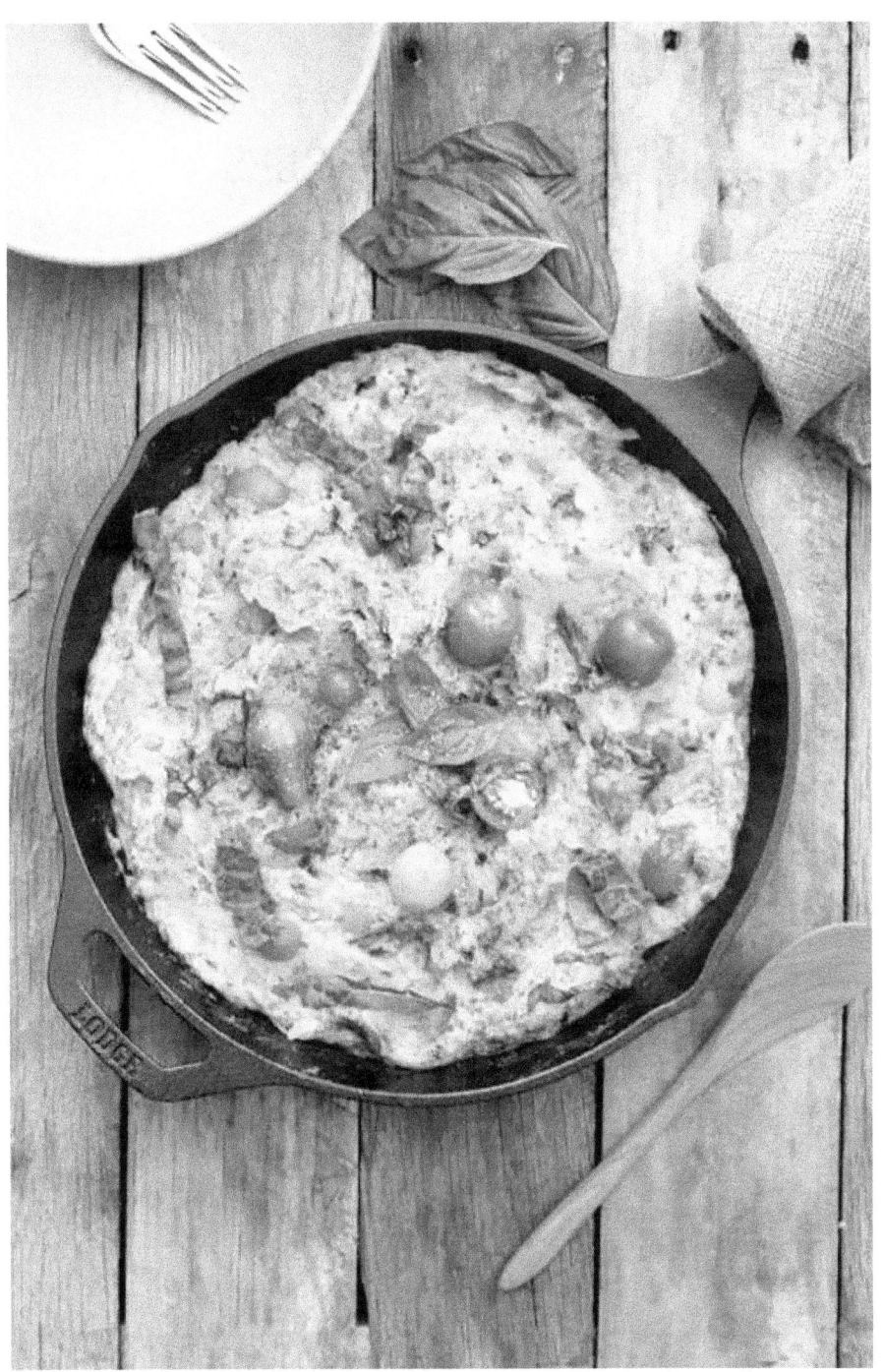

ITALIAN SPICE-RUBBED PORK ROAST WITH VEGETABLES

PREP: 20 minutes ROAST: 2 hours 25 minutes STAND: 10 minutes MAKES: 8 servings

"FRESH IS BEST" IS A GOOD MANTRA TO FOLLOW WHEN IT COMES TO COOKING MOST OF THE TIME. HOWEVER, DRIED HERBS WORK VERY WELL IN RUBS FOR MEATS. WHEN HERBS ARE DRIED, THEIR FLAVORS ARE CONCENTRATED. WHEN THEY COME INTO CONTACT WITH MOISTURE FROM THE MEAT, THEY RELEASE THEIR FLAVORS INTO IT, AS IN THIS ITALIAN-STYLE ROAST FLAVORED WITH PARSLEY, FENNEL, OREGANO, GARLIC, AND SPICY CRUSHED RED PEPPER.

2 tablespoons dried parsley, crushed

2 tablespoons fennel seeds, crushed

4 teaspoons dried oregano, crushed

1 teaspoon freshly ground black pepper

½ teaspoon crushed red pepper

4 cloves garlic, minced

1 4-pound bone-in pork shoulder roast

1 to 2 tablespoons olive oil

1¼ cups water

2 medium onions, peeled and cut into wedges

1 large fennel bulb, trimmed, cored, and cut into wedges

2 pounds Brussels sprouts

1. Preheat oven to 325°F. In a small bowl combine parsley, fennel seeds, oregano, black pepper, crushed red pepper, and garlic; set aside. Untie pork roast if necessary. Trim fat from meat. Rub the meat on all sides with the seasoning mixture. If desired, retie roast to hold it together.

2. In a Dutch oven heat oil over medium-high heat. Brown meat on all sides in the hot oil. Drain off fat. Pour the water into Dutch oven around roast. Roast, uncovered, for 1½ hours. Arrange onions and fennel around pork roast. Cover and roast for 30 minutes more.

3. Meanwhile, trim Brussels sprouts stems and remove any wilted outer leaves. Cut Brussels sprouts in half. Add Brussels sprouts to Dutch oven, arranging them over other vegetables. Cover and roast for 30 to 35 minutes more or until vegetables and meat are tender. Transfer meat to a serving platter and cover with foil. Let stand for 15 minutes before slicing. Toss vegetables with pan juices to coat. Using a slotted spoon, remove vegetables to the serving platter or a bowl; cover to keep warm.

4. Using a large spoon, skim fat from pan juices. Pour remaining pan juices through a sieve. Slice pork, removing the bone. Serve meat with vegetables and pan juices.

SLOW COOKER PORK MOLE

PREP: 20 minutes SLOW COOK: 8 to 10 hours (low) or 4 to 5 hours (high) MAKES: 8 servings

WITH CUMIN, CORIANDER, OREGANO, TOMATOES, ALMONDS, RAISINS, CHILE, AND CHOCOLATE, THIS RICH AND SPICY SAUCE HAS A LOT GOING ON—IN A VERY GOOD WAY. IT'S AN IDEAL MEAL TO START IN THE MORNING BEFORE YOU HEAD OUT FOR THE DAY. WHEN YOU COME HOME, DINNER IS NEARLY DONE—AND YOUR HOUSE SMELLS AMAZING.

- 1 3-pound boneless pork shoulder roast
- 1 cup coarsely chopped onion
- 3 cloves garlic, sliced
- 1½ cups Beef Bone Broth (see recipe), Chicken Bone Broth (see recipe), or no-salt-added beef or chicken broth
- 1 tablespoon ground cumin
- 1 tablespoon ground coriander
- 2 teaspoons dried oregano, crushed
- 1 15-ounce can diced no-salt-added tomatoes, drained
- 1 6-ounce can no-salt-added tomato paste
- ½ cup slivered almonds, toasted (see tip)
- ¼ cup unsulfured golden raisins or currants
- 2 ounces unsweetened chocolate (such as Scharffen Berger 99% cacao bar), coarsely chopped
- 1 dried whole ancho or chipotle chile pepper
- 2 4-inch cinnamon sticks
- ¼ cup snipped fresh cilantro
- 1 avocado, peeled, seeded, and thinly sliced
- 1 lime, cut into wedges
- ⅓ cup toasted unsalted green pumpkin seeds (optional) (see tip)

1. Trim fat from pork roast. If necessary, cut meat to fit a 5- to 6-quart slow cooker; set aside.

2. In the slow cooker combine onion and garlic. In a 2-cup glass measuring cup stir together Beef Bone Broth, cumin, coriander, and oregano; pour into cooker. Stir in diced tomatoes, tomato paste, almonds, raisins, chocolate, dried chile pepper, and cinnamon sticks. Place meat in cooker. Spoon some of the tomato mixture over the top. Cover and cook on low-heat setting for 8 to 10 hours or on high-heat setting for 4 to 5 hours or until pork is tender.

3. Transfer pork to a cutting board; cool slightly. Using two forks, pull meat apart into shreds. Cover meat with foil and set aside.

4. Remove and discard dried chile pepper and cinnamon sticks. Using a large spoon, skim fat from tomato mixture. Transfer the tomato mixture to a blender or food processor. Cover and blend or process until almost smooth. Return pulled pork and sauce into slow cooker. Keep warm on low-heat setting until serving time, up to 2 hours.

5. Just before serving, stir in cilantro. Serve mole in bowls and garnish with avocado slices, lime wedges, and, if desired, pumpkin seeds.

CARAWAY-SPICED PORK AND SQUASH STEW

PREP: 30 minutes COOK: 1 hour MAKES: 4 servings

PEPPERY MUSTARD GREENS AND BUTTERNUT SQUASH ADD VIBRANT COLOR AND A WHOLE HOST OF VITAMINS—AS WELL AS FIBER AND FOLIC ACID—TO THIS STEW SPICED WITH EASTERN EUROPEAN FLAVORS.

1 1¼- to 1½-pound pork shoulder roast

1 tablespoon paprika

1 tablespoon caraway seeds, finely crushed

2 teaspoons dry mustard

¼ teaspoon cayenne pepper

2 tablespoon refined coconut oil

8 ounces fresh button mushrooms, thinly sliced

2 stalks celery, cut crosswise into 1-inch slices

1 small red onion, cut into thin wedges

6 cloves garlic, minced

5 cups Chicken Bone Broth (see recipe) or no-salt-added chicken broth

2 cups cubed, peeled butternut squash

3 cups coarsely chopped, trimmed mustard greens or green cabbage

2 tablespoons snipped fresh sage

¼ cup fresh lemon juice

1. Trim fat from pork. Cut pork into 1½-inch cubes; place in a large bowl. In a small bowl combine paprika, caraway seeds, dry mustard, and cayenne pepper. Sprinkle over pork, tossing to coat evenly.

2. In a 4- to 5-quart Dutch oven heat coconut oil over medium heat. Add half of the meat; cook until browned, stirring

occasionally. Remove meat from the pan. Repeat with the remaining meat. Set meat aside.

3. Add mushrooms, celery, red onion, and garlic to Dutch oven. Cook for 5 minutes, stirring occasionally. Return meat to the Dutch oven. Carefully add Chicken Bone Broth. Bring to boiling; reduce heat. Cover and simmer for 45 minutes. Stir in squash. Cover and simmer for 10 to 15 minutes more or until pork and squash are tender. Stir in mustard greens and sage. Cook for 2 to 3 minutes or until greens are just tender. Stir in lemon juice.

FRUIT-STUFFED TOP LOIN ROAST WITH BRANDY SAUCE

PREP: 30 minutes COOK: 10 minutes ROAST: 1 hour 15 minutes STAND: 15 minutes
MAKES: 8 to 10 servings

THIS ELEGANT ROAST IS PERFECT FOR A SPECIAL OCCASION OR FAMILY GATHERING—PARTICULARLY IN THE FALL. ITS FLAVORS—APPLES, NUTMEG, DRIED FRUIT, AND PECANS—CAPTURE THE ESSENCE OF THAT SEASON. SERVE IT WITH MASHED SWEET POTATOES AND BLUEBERRY AND ROASTED BEET KALE SALAD (SEE RECIPE).

ROAST
- 1 tablespoon olive oil
- 2 cups chopped, peeled Granny Smith apples (about 2 medium)
- 1 shallot, finely chopped
- 1 tablespoon snipped fresh thyme
- ¾ teaspoon freshly ground black pepper
- ⅛ teaspoon ground nutmeg
- ½ cup snipped unsulfured dried apricots
- ¼ cup chopped pecans, toasted (see tip)
- 1 cup Chicken Bone Broth (see recipe) or no-salt-added chicken broth
- 1 3-pound boneless pork top loin roast (single loin)

BRANDY SAUCE
- 2 tablespoons apple cider
- 2 tablespoons brandy
- 1 teaspoon Dijon-Style Mustard (see recipe)
- Freshly ground black pepper

1. For the stuffing, in a large skillet heat olive oil over medium heat. Add apples, shallot, thyme, ¼ teaspoon of the pepper, and nutmeg; cook for 2 to 4 minutes or until

apples and shallot are tender and light golden, stirring occasionally. Stir in apricots, pecans, and 1 tablespoon of the broth. Cook, uncovered, for 1 minute to soften apricots. Remove from heat and set aside.

2. Preheat oven to 325°F. Butterfly the pork roast by making a lengthwise cut down the center of the roast, cutting to within ½ inch of the other side. Spread the roast open. Place the knife in the V cut, facing it horizontally toward one side of the V, and cut to within ½ inch of the side. Repeat on the other side of the V. Spread the roast open and cover with plastic wrap. Working from the center to the edges, pound the roast with a meat mallet until it is about ¾ inch thick. Remove and discard plastic wrap. Spread the stuffing over the top of the roast. Starting from a short side, roll the roast into a spiral. Tie with 100%-cotton kitchen string in several places to hold the roast together. Sprinkle roast with the remaining ½ teaspoon pepper.

3. Place roast on a rack in a shallow roasting pan. Insert an oven-going thermometer into the center of the roast (not in the stuffing). Roast, uncovered, for 1 hour 15 minutes to 1 hour 30 minutes or until thermometer registers 145°F. Remove roast and cover loosely with foil; let stand for 15 minutes before slicing.

4. Meanwhile, for Brandy Sauce, stir the remaining broth and apple cider into drippings in pan, whisking to scrape up browned bits. Strain drippings into a medium saucepan. Bring to boiling; cook about 4 minutes or until sauce is reduced by one-third. Stir in brandy and Dijon-Style

Mustard. Season to taste with additional pepper. Serve sauce with the pork roast.

PORCHETTA-STYLE PORK ROAST

PREP: 15 minutes MARINATE: overnight STAND: 40 minutes ROAST: 1 hour MAKES: 6 servings

TRADITIONAL ITALIAN PORCHETTA (SOMETIMES SPELLED PORKETTA IN AMERICAN ENGLISH) IS A BONELESS SUCKLING PIG STUFFED WITH GARLIC, FENNEL, PEPPER, AND HERBS SUCH AS SAGE OR ROSEMARY, THEN PUT ON A SPIT AND ROASTED OVER WOOD. IT'S ALSO USUALLY HEAVILY SALTED. THIS PALEO VERSION IS SIMPLIFIED AND VERY TASTY. SUBSTITUTE FRESH ROSEMARY FOR THE SAGE, IF YOU LIKE, OR USE A BLEND OF THE TWO HERBS.

1 2- to 3-pound boneless pork loin roast
2 tablespoons fennel seeds
1 teaspoon black peppercorns
½ teaspoon crushed red pepper
6 cloves garlic, minced
1 tablespoon finely shredded orange peel
1 tablespoon snipped fresh sage
3 tablespoon olive oil
½ cup dry white wine
½ cup Chicken Bone Broth (see recipe) or no-salt-added chicken broth

1. Remove pork roast from refrigerator; let stand at room temperature for 30 minutes. Meanwhile, in a small skillet toast fennel seeds over medium heat, stirring frequently, about 3 minutes or until dark in color and fragrant; cool. Transfer to a spice mill or clean coffee grinder. Add peppercorns and crushed red pepper. Grind to medium-fine consistency. (Do not grind to a powder.)

2. Preheat oven to 325°F. In a small bowl combine ground spices, garlic, orange peel, sage, and olive oil to make a paste. Place pork roast on a rack in a small roasting pan. Rub mixture all over pork. (If desired, place seasoned pork in a 9×13×2-inch glass baking dish. Cover with with plastic wrap and refrigerate overnight to marinate. Transfer meat to a roasting pan before cooking and let stand at room temperature for 30 minutes before cooking.)

3. Roast pork for 1 to 1½ hours or until an instant-read thermometer inserted into center of roast registers 145°F. Transfer roast to a cutting board and cover loosely with foil. Let stand for 10 to 15 minutes before slicing.

4. Meanwhile, pour pan juices into a glass measuring cup. Skim fat from top; set aside. Place roasting pan on stovetop burner. Pour wine and Chicken Bone Broth into pan. Bring to boiling over medium-high heat, stirring to scrape up any browned bits. Boil about 4 minutes or until mixture is slightly reduced. Whisk in reserved pan juices; strain. Slice pork and serve with sauce.

TOMATILLO-BRAISED PORK LOIN

PREP: 40 minutes BROIL: 10 minutes COOK: 20 minutes ROAST: 40 minutes STAND: 10 minutes MAKES: 6 to 8 servings

TOMATILLOS HAVE A STICKY, SAPPY COATING UNDER THEIR PAPER SKINS. AFTER YOU REMOVE THE SKINS, GIVE THEM A QUICK RINSE UNDER RUNNING WATER AND THEY ARE READY TO USE.

1 pound tomatillos, husked, stemmed, and rinsed
4 serrano chiles, stemmed, seeded, and halved (see tip)
2 jalapeños, stemmed, seeded, and halved (see tip)
1 large yellow sweet pepper, stemmed, seeded, and halved
1 large orange sweet pepper, stemmed, seeded, and halved
2 tablespoons olive oil
1 2- to 2½-pound boneless pork loin roast
1 large yellow onion, peeled, halved, and thinly sliced
4 cloves garlic, minced
¾ cup water
¼ cup fresh lime juice
¼ cup snipped fresh cilantro

1. Preheat broiler to high. Line a baking sheet with foil. Arrange tomatillos, serrano chiles, jalapeños, and sweet peppers on prepared baking sheet. Broil vegetables 4 inches from heat until well charred, turning tomatillos occasionally and removing vegetables as they become charred, about 10 to 15 minutes. Place serranos, jalapeños, and tomatillos in a bowl. Place sweet peppers on a plate. Set vegetables aside to cool.

2. In a large skillet heat oil over medium-high heat until it shimmers. Pat pork roast dry with clean paper towels and add to skillet. Cook until well browned on all sides,

turning roast to brown evenly. Transfer roast to a platter. Reduce heat to medium. Add onion to skillet; cook and stir for 5 to 6 minutes or until golden. Add garlic; cook for 1 minute more. Remove skillet from heat.

3. Preheat oven to 350°F. For tomatillo sauce, in a food processor or blender combine tomatillos, serranos, and jalapeños. Cover and blend or process until smooth; add to onion in skillet. Return skillet to heat. Bring to boiling; cook for 4 to 5 minutes or until mixture is dark and thick. Stir in the water, lime juice, and cilantro.

4. Spread tomatillo sauce in a shallow roasting pan or 3-quart rectangular baking dish. Place pork roast in the sauce. Cover tightly with foil. Roast for 40 to 45 minutes or until an instant-read thermometer inserted into the center of the roast reads 140°F.

5. Cut sweet peppers into strips. Stir into the tomatillo sauce in pan. Tent loosely with foil; let stand for 10 minutes. Slice meat; stir sauce. Serve sliced pork topped generously with tomatillo sauce.

APRICOT-STUFFED PORK TENDERLOIN

PREP: 20 minutes ROAST: 45 minutes STAND: 5 minutes MAKES: 2 to 3 servings

- 2 medium fresh apricots, coarsely chopped
- 2 tablespoons unsulfured raisins
- 2 tablespoons chopped walnuts
- 2 teaspoons grated fresh ginger
- ¼ teaspoon ground cardamom
- 1 12-ounce pork tenderloin
- 1 tablespoon olive oil
- 1 tablespoon Dijon-Style Mustard (see recipe)
- ¼ teaspoon black pepper

1. Preheat oven to 375°F. Line a baking sheet with foil; place a roasting rack on the baking sheet.

2. In a small bowl stir together the apricots, raisins, walnuts, ginger, and cardamom.

3. Make a lengthwise cut down the center of the pork, cutting to within ½ inch of the other side. Butterfly it open. Place the pork between two layers of plastic wrap. Using the flat side of a meat mallet, lightly pound meat until about ⅓ inch thick. Fold in the tail end to make an even rectangle. Lightly pound meat to make even thickness.

4. Spread the apricot mixture over the pork. Beginning at the narrow end, roll up the pork. Tie with 100%-cotton kitchen string, first in the center, then at 1-inch intervals. Place roast on the rack.

5. Stir together the olive oil and Dijon-Style Mustard; brush over the roast. Sprinkle roast with pepper. Roast for 45 to

55 minutes or until an instant-read thermometer inserted into center of roast registers 140°F. Let stand for 5 to 10 minutes before slicing.

HERB-CRUSTED PORK TENDERLOIN WITH CRISPY GARLIC OIL

PREP: 15 minutes ROAST: 30 minutes COOK: 8 minutes STAND: 5 minutes MAKES: 6 servings

⅓ cup Dijon-Style Mustard (see recipe)
¼ cup snipped fresh parsley
2 tablespoons snipped fresh thyme
1 tablespoon snipped fresh rosemary
½ teaspoon black pepper
2 12-ounce pork tenderloins
½ cup olive oil
¼ cup minced fresh garlic
¼ to 1 teaspoon crushed red pepper

1. Preheat oven to 450°F. Line a baking sheet with foil; place a roasting rack on the baking sheet.

2. In a small bowl stir together the mustard, parsley, thyme, rosemary, and black pepper to make a paste. Spread the mustard-herb mixture over the top and sides of the pork. Transfer pork to the roasting rack. Place roast in the oven; decrease temperature to 375°F. Roast for 30 to 35 minutes or until an instant-read thermometer inserted into center of roast registers 140°F. Let stand for 5 to 10 minutes before slicing.

3. Meanwhile, for garlic oil, in a small saucepan combine the olive oil and garlic. Cook over medium-low heat for 8 to 10 minutes or until garlic is golden and begins to crisp (do not let garlic burn). Remove from heat; stir in crushed red pepper. Slice pork; spoon garlic oil over the slices before serving.

INDIAN-SPICED PORK WITH COCONUT PAN SAUCE

START TO FINISH: 20 minutes MAKES: 2 servings

3 teaspoons curry powder
2 teaspoons salt-free garam masala
1 teaspoon ground cumin
1 teaspoon ground coriander
1 12-ounce pork tenderloin
1 tablespoon olive oil
½ cup natural coconut milk (such as Nature's Way brand)
¼ cup snipped fresh cilantro
2 tablespoons snipped fresh mint

1. In a small bowl stir together 2 teaspoons of the curry powder, garam masala, cumin, and coriander. Slice pork into ½-inch-thick slices; sprinkle with spices. .

2. In a large skillet heat olive oil over medium heat. Add pork slices to skillet; cook for 7 minutes, turning once. Remove pork from skillet; cover to keep warm. For sauce, add coconut milk and the remaining 1 teaspoon curry powder to the skillet, stirring to scrape up any bits. Simmer for 2 to 3 minutes. Stir in cilantro and mint. Add pork; cook until heated through, spooning sauce over the pork.

PORK SCALOPPINI WITH SPICED APPLES AND CHESTNUTS

PREP: 20 minutes COOK: 15 minutes MAKES: 4 servings

2 12-ounce pork tenderloins
1 tablespoon onion powder
1 tablespoon garlic powder
½ teaspoon black pepper
2 to 4 tablespoons olive oil
2 Fuji or Pink Lady apples, peeled, cored, and coarsely chopped
¼ cup finely chopped shallots
¾ teaspoon ground cinnamon
⅛ teaspoon ground cloves
⅛ teaspoon ground nutmeg
½ cup Chicken Bone Broth (see recipe) or no-salt added chicken broth
2 tablespoons fresh lemon juice
½ cup peeled roasted chestnuts, chopped,* or chopped pecans
1 tablespoon snipped fresh sage

1. Cut the tenderloins into ½-inch- thick slices on a bias. Place pork slices between two sheets of plastic wrap. Using the flat side of a meat mallet, pound until thin. Sprinkle slices with onion powder, garlic powder, and black pepper.

2. In a large skillet heat 2 tablespoons olive oil over medium heat. Cook pork, in batches, for 3 to 4 minutes, turning once and adding oil if necessary. Transfer pork to a plate; cover and keep warm.

3. Increase heat to medium-high. Add the apples, shallots, cinnamon, cloves, and nutmeg. Cook and stir for 3 minutes. Stir in Chicken Bone Broth and lemon juice.

Cover and cook for 5 minutes. Remove from heat; stir in the chestnuts and sage. Serve apple mixture over pork.

*Note: To roast chestnuts, preheat oven to 400°F. Cut an X in one side of the chestnut shell. This will let the shell loosen as it cooks. Place chestnuts on a baking pan and roast for 30 minutes or until the shell pulls apart from the nut and the nuts are tender. Wrap the roasted chestnuts in a clean kitchen towel. Peel shells and skin from the yellow-white nut.

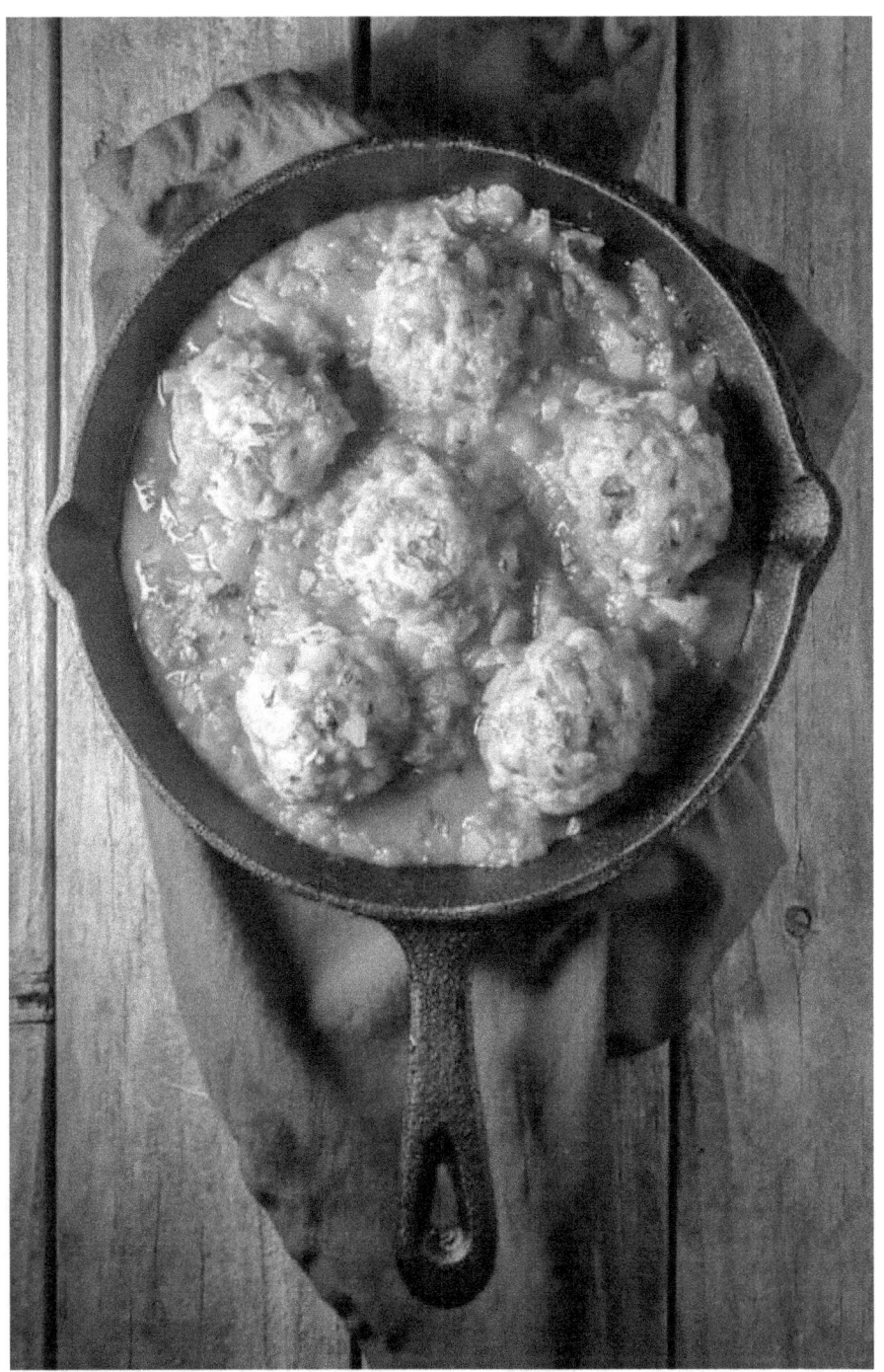

PORK FAJITA STIR-FRY

PREP: 20 minutes COOK: 22 minutes MAKES: 4 servings

1 pound pork tenderloin, cut into 2-inch strips
3 tablespoons salt-free fajita seasoning or Mexican Seasoning (see recipe)
2 tablespoons olive oil
1 small onion, thinly sliced
½ of a red sweet pepper, seeded and thinly sliced
½ of an orange sweet pepper, seeded and thinly sliced
1 jalapeño, stemmed and thinly sliced (see tip) (optional)
½ teaspoon cumin seeds
1 cup thinly sliced fresh mushrooms
3 tablespoons fresh lime juice
½ cup snipped fresh cilantro
1 avocado, seeded, peeled, and diced
Desired salsa (see recipes)

1. Sprinkle the pork with 2 tablespoons fajita seasoning. In an extra-large skillet heat 1 tablespoon of the oil over medium-high heat. Add half the pork; cook and stir about 5 minutes or until no longer pink. Transfer meat to a bowl and cover to keep warm. Repeat with remaining oil and pork.

2. Turn heat to medium. Add the remaining 1 tablespoon fajita seasoning, onion, sweet peppers, jalapeño, and cumin. Cook and stir about 10 minutes or until vegetables are tender. Return all the meat and accumulated juices to skillet. Stir in mushrooms and lime juice. Cook until heated through. Remove skillet from heat; stir in the cilantro. Serve with avocado and desired salsa.

PORK TENDERLOIN WITH PORT AND PRUNES

PREP: 10 minutes ROAST: 12 minutes STAND: 5 minutes MAKES: 4 servings

PORT IS A FORTIFIED WINE, WHICH MEANS IT HAS A SPIRIT SIMILAR TO BRANDY ADDED TO IT TO STOP THE FERMENTATION PROCESS. THIS MEANS THERE IS MORE RESIDUAL SUGAR IN IT THAN RED TABLE WINE AND CONSEQUENTLY IT HAS A SWEETER TASTE. IT ISN'T SOMETHING YOU WANT TO DRINK EVERY DAY, BUT A LITTLE BIT USED IN COOKING ONCE IN A WHILE IS FINE.

2 12-ounce pork tenderloins
2½ teaspoons ground coriander
¼ teaspoon black pepper
2 tablespoons olive oil
1 shallot, sliced
½ cup port wine
½ cup Chicken Bone Broth (see recipe) or no-salt-added chicken broth
20 pitted unsulfured dried plums (prunes)
½ teaspoon crushed red pepper
2 teaspoons snipped fresh tarragon

1. Preheat oven to 400°F. Sprinkle pork with 2 teaspoons of the coriander and the black pepper.

2. In a large ovenproof skillet heat olive oil over medium-high heat. Add tenderloins to skillet. Cook until browned on all sides, turning to brown evenly, about 8 minutes. Place skillet in oven. Roast, uncovered, about 12 minutes or until an instant-read thermometer inserted into center of roasts registers 140°F. Transfer tenderloins to a cutting

board. Cover loosely with aluminum foil and let stand for 5 minutes.

3. Meanwhile, for sauce, drain fat from skillet, reserving 1 tablespoon. Cook shallot in the reserved drippings in skillet over medium heat about 3 minutes or until browned and tender. Add port to skillet. Bring to boiling, stirring to scrape up any browned bits. Add Chicken Bone Broth, dried plums, crushed red pepper, and the remaining ½ teaspoon coriander. Cook over medium-high heat to reduce slightly, about 1 to 2 minutes. Stir in tarragon.

4. Slice pork and serve with prunes and sauce.

MOO SHU-STYLE PORK IN LETTUCE CUPS WITH QUICK PICKLED VEGETABLES

START TO FINISH: 45 minutes MAKES: 4 servings

IF YOU'VE HAD A TRADITIONAL MOO SHU DISH IN A CHINESE RESTAURANT, YOU KNOW IT IS A SAVORY MEAT AND VEGETABLE FILLING EATEN IN THIN PANCAKES WITH A SWEET PLUM OR HOISIN SAUCE. THIS LIGHTER AND FRESHER PALEO VERSION FEATURES PORK, CHINESE CABBAGE, AND SHIITAKE MUSHROOMS STIR-FRIED IN GINGER AND GARLIC AND ENJOYED IN LETTUCE WRAPS WITH CRUNCHY PICKLED VEGETABLES.

PICKLED VEGETABLES
- 1 cup julienne-cut carrots
- 1 cup julienne-cut daikon radish
- ¼ cup slivered red onion
- 1 cup unsweetened apple juice
- ½ cup cider vinegar

PORK
- 2 tablespoons olive oil or refined coconut oil
- 3 eggs, lightly beaten
- 8 ounces pork loin, cut into 2×½-inch strips
- 2 teaspoons minced fresh ginger
- 4 cloves garlic, minced
- 2 cups thinly sliced napa cabbage
- 1 cup thinly sliced shiitake mushrooms
- ¼ cup thinly sliced scallions
- 8 Boston lettuce leaves

1. For quick pickled vegetables, in a large bowl toss together the carrots, daikon, and onion. For brine, in a saucepan heat the apple juice and vinegar just until steam rises. Pour the brine over the vegetables in bowl; cover and chill until ready to serve.

2. In a large skillet heat 1 tablespoon of the oil over medium-high heat. Using a whisk, lightly beat eggs. Add eggs to skillet; cook, without stirring, until set on the bottom, about 3 minutes. Using a flexible spatula, carefully turn the egg over and cook on the other side. Slide the egg out of the pan onto a platter.

3. Return the skillet to heat; add the remaining 1 tablespoon oil. Add the pork strips, ginger, and garlic. Cook and stir over medium-high heat about 4 minutes or until pork is no longer pink. Add the cabbage and mushrooms; cook and stir about 4 minutes or until cabbage wilts, mushrooms soften, and pork is cooked through. Remove skillet from heat. Cut the cooked egg into strips. Gently stir egg strips and scallions into pork mixture. Serve in lettuce leaves and top with pickled vegetables.

PORK CHOPS WITH MACADAMIAS, SAGE, FIGS, AND MASHED SWEET POTATOES

PREP: 15 minutes COOK: 25 minutes MAKES: 4 servings

PAIRED WITH MASHED SWEET POTATOES, THESE JUICY SAGE-TOPPED CHOPS MAKE A PERFECT FALL MEAL—AND ONE THAT'S QUICK TO FIX, MAKING IT A PERFECT FOR A BUSY WEEKNIGHT.

4 boneless pork loin chops, cut 1¼ inches thick
3 tablespoons snipped fresh sage
¼ teaspoon black pepper
3 tablespoons macadamia nut oil
2 pounds sweet potatoes, peeled and cut into 1-inch pieces
¾ cup chopped macadamia nuts
½ cup chopped dried figs
⅓ cup Beef Bone Broth (see recipe) or no-salt-added beef broth
1 tablespoon fresh lemon juice

1. Sprinkle both sides of pork chops with 2 tablespoons of the sage and the pepper; rub in with your fingers. In a large skillet heat 2 tablespoons of the oil over medium heat. Add chops to skillet; cook for 15 to 20 minutes or until done (145°F), turning once halfway through cooking. Transfer chops to a plate; cover to keep warm.

2. Meanwhile, in a large saucepan combine sweet potatoes and enough water to cover. Bring to boiling; reduce heat. Cover and simmer for 10 to 15 minutes or until potatoes are tender. Drain potatoes. Add the remaining tablespoon macadamia oil to potatoes and mash until creamy; keep warm.

3. For sauce, add macadamia nuts to skillet; cook over medium heat just until toasted. Add dried figs and the remaining 1 tablespoon sage; cook for 30 seconds. Add Beef Bone Broth and lemon juice to skillet, stirring to scrape up any browned bits. Spoon sauce over pork chops and serve with mashed sweet potatoes.

SKILLET-ROASTED ROSEMARY-LAVENDER PORK CHOPS WITH GRAPES AND TOASTED WALNUTS

PREP: 10 minutes COOK: 6 minutes ROAST: 25 minutes MAKES: 4 servings

ROASTING THE GRAPES ALONG WITH THE PORK CHOPS INTENSIFIES THEIR FLAVOR AND SWEETNESS. ALONG WITH THE CRUNCHY TOASTED WALNUTS AND A SPRINKLING OF FRESH ROSEMARY, THEY MAKE A WONDERFUL TOPPING FOR THESE HEARTY CHOPS.

2 tablespoons snipped fresh rosemary
1 tablespoon snipped fresh lavender
½ teaspoon garlic powder
½ teaspoon black pepper
4 pork loin chops, cut 1¼ inches thick (about 3 pounds)
1 tablespoon olive oil
1 large shallot, thinly sliced
1½ cups red and/or green seedless grapes
½ cup dry white wine
¾ cup coarsely chopped walnuts
Snipped fresh rosemary

1. Preheat oven to 375°F. In a small bowl combine 2 tablespoons rosemary, lavender, garlic powder, and pepper. Rub herb mixture evenly into pork chops. In an extra-large ovenproof skillet heat olive oil over medium heat. Add chops to skillet; cook for 6 to 8 minutes or until browned on both sides. Transfer chops to a plate; cover with foil.

2. Add the shallot to the skillet. Cook and stir over medium heat for 1 minute. Add grapes and wine. Cook about 2 minutes more, stirring to scrape up any browned bits. Return pork chops to skillet. Place the skillet in the oven; roast for 25 to 30 minutes or until chops are done (145°F).

3. Meanwhile, spread the walnuts in a shallow baking pan. Add to oven with chops. Roast about 8 minutes or until toasted, stirring once to toast evenly.

4. To serve, top pork chops with grapes and toasted walnuts. Sprinkle with additional fresh rosemary.

PORK CHOPS ALLA FIORENTINA WITH GRILLED BROCCOLI RABE

PREP: 20 minutes GRILL: 20 minutes MARINATE: 3 minutes MAKES: 4 servings PHOTO

"ALLA FIORENTINA" ESSENTIALLY MEANS "IN THE STYLE OF FLORENCE." THIS RECIPE IS STYLED AFTER *BISTECCA ALLA FIORENTINA*, A TUSCAN T-BONE GRILLED OVER A WOOD FIRE WITH THE SIMPLEST FLAVORINGS—USUALLY JUST OLIVE OIL, SALT, BLACK PEPPER, AND A SQUEEZE OF FRESH LEMON TO FINISH.

1 pound broccoli rabe
1 tablespoon olive oil
4 6- to 8-ounce bone-in pork loin chops, cut 1½ to 2 inches thick
Coarsely ground black pepper
1 lemon
4 cloves garlic, thinly sliced
2 tablespoons snipped fresh rosemary
6 fresh sage leaves, chopped
1 teaspoon crushed red pepper flakes (or to taste)
½ cup olive oil

1. In a large saucepan blanch the broccoli rabe in boiling water for 1 minute. Immediately transfer to a bowl of ice water. When cool, drain the broccoli rabe on a paper towel-lined baking sheet, blotting as dry as possible with additional paper towels. Remove paper towels from baking sheet. Drizzle the broccoli rabe with 1 tablespoon olive oil, tossing to coat; set aside until ready to grill.

2. Sprinkle both sides of the pork chops with coarsely ground pepper; set aside. Using a vegetable peeler, remove strips

of peel from lemon (save lemon for another use). Scatter lemon peel strips, sliced garlic, rosemary, sage, and crushed red pepper on a large serving platter; set aside.

3. For a charcoal grill, move most hot coals to one side of the grill, leaving some coals under the other side of the grill. Sear the chops directly over the hot coals for 2 to 3 minutes or until a brown crust forms. Turn the chops over and sear on the second side for 2 minutes more. Move the chops to the other side of the grill. Cover and grill for 10 to 15 minutes or until done (145°F). (For a gas grill, preheat grill; reduce heat on one side of grill to medium. Sear chops as directed above over high heat. Move to medium heat side of grill; continue as directed above.)

4. Transfer the chops to the platter. Drizzle chops with the ½ cup olive oil, turning to coat both sides. Let the chops marinate for 3 to 5 minutes before serving, turning once or twice to infuse the meat with the flavors of the lemon peel, garlic, and herbs.

5. While the chops rest, grill the broccoli rabe to char lightly and warm through. Arrange broccoli rabe on the platter with the pork chops; spoon some of the marinade over each chop and broccoli rabe before serving.

ESCAROLE-STUFFED PORK CHOPS

PREP: 20 minutes COOK: 9 minutes MAKES: 4 servings

ESCAROLE CAN BE EATEN AS A SALAD GREEN OR LIGHTLY SAUTÉED WITH GARLIC IN OLIVE OIL FOR A QUICK SIDE DISH. HERE, COMBINED WITH OLIVE OIL, GARLIC, BLACK PEPPER, CRUSHED RED PEPPER, AND LEMON, IT MAKES A BEAUTIFUL BRIGHT-GREEN FILLING FOR JUICY PAN-SEARED PORK CHOPS.

4 6- to 8-ounce bone-in pork chops, cut ¾ inch thick

½ of a medium head escarole, finely chopped

4 tablespoons olive oil

1 tablespoon fresh lemon juice

¼ teaspoon black pepper

¼ teaspoon crushed red pepper

2 large cloves garlic, minced

Olive oil

1 tablespoon snipped fresh sage

¼ teaspoon black pepper

⅓ cup dry white wine

1. Using a paring knife, cut a deep pocket, about 2 inches wide, into the curved side of each pork chop; set aside.

2. In a large bowl combine escarole, 2 tablespoons of the olive oil, lemon juice, ¼ teaspoon black pepper, crushed red pepper, and garlic. Stuff each chop with one-fourth of the mixture. Brush chops with olive oil. Sprinkle with sage and ¼ teaspoon ground black pepper.

3. In an extra-large skillet heat remaining 2 tablespoons olive oil over medium-high heat. Sear pork for 4 minutes on each side until golden brown. Transfer chops to a plate.

Add wine to skillet, scraping up any browned bits. Reduce pan juices for 1 minute.

4. Drizzle chops with pan juices before serving.

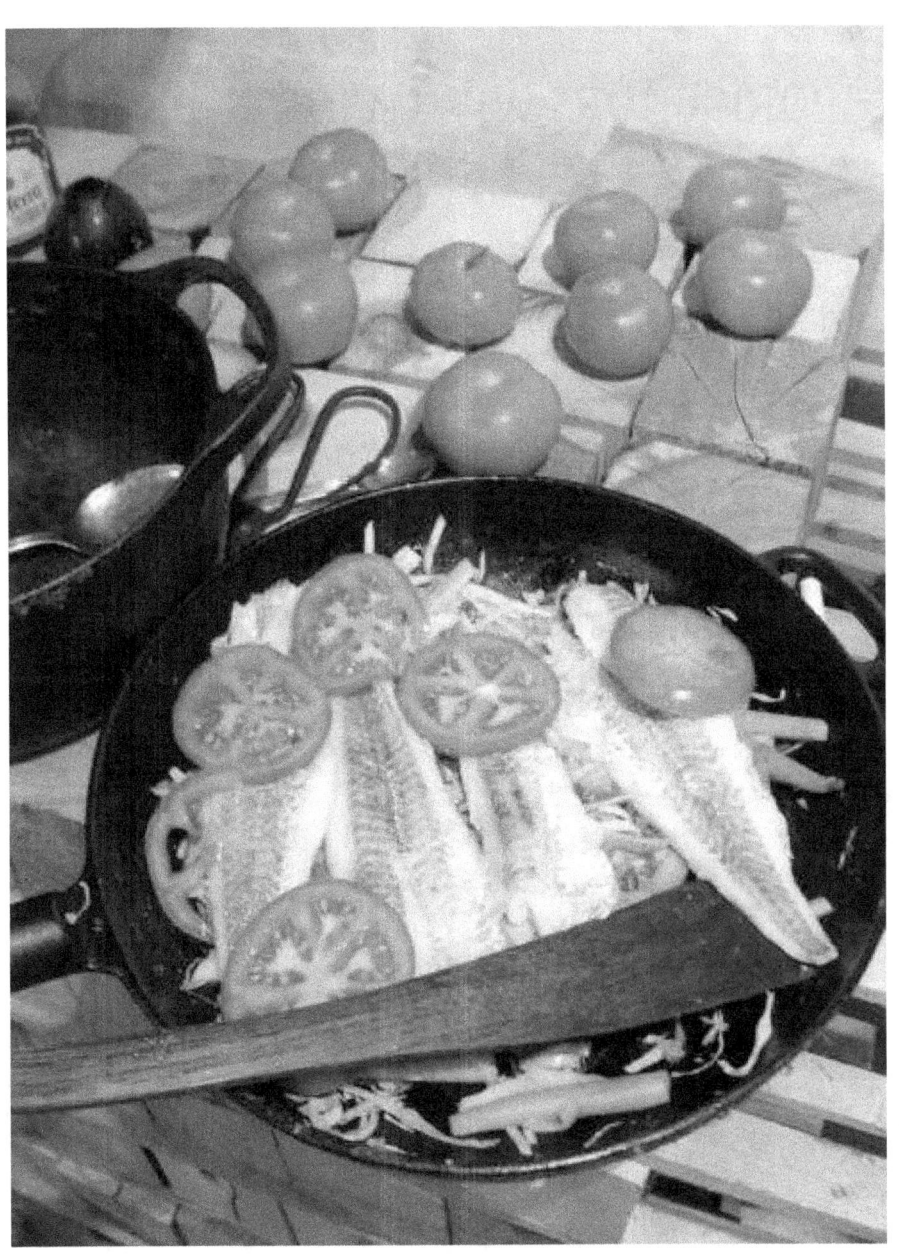

PORK CHOPS WITH A DIJON-PECAN CRUST

PREP: 15 minutes COOK: 6 minutes BAKE: 3 minutes MAKES: 4 servings PHOTO

THESE MUSTARD-AND-NUT-CRUSTED CHOPS COULDN'T BE SIMPLER TO MAKE—AND THE TASTE PAY-OFF FAR EXCEEDS THE EFFORT. TRY THEM WITH CINNAMON-ROASTED BUTTERNUT SQUASH (SEE RECIPE), NEO-CLASSIC WALDORF SALAD (SEE RECIPE), OR BRUSSELS SPROUTS AND APPLE SALAD (SEE RECIPE).

⅓ cup finely chopped pecans, toasted (see tip)
1 tablespoon snipped fresh sage
3 tablespoons olive oil
4 bone-in center-cut pork chops, about 1 inch thick (about 2 pounds total)
½ teaspoon black pepper
2 tablespoons olive oil
3 tablespoons Dijon-Style Mustard (see recipe)

1. Preheat oven to 400°F. In a small bowl combine pecans, sage, and 1 tablespoon of the olive oil.

2. Sprinkle pork chops with pepper. In a large ovenproof skillet heat the remaining 2 tablespoons olive oil over high heat. Add chops; cook about 6 minutes or until browned on both sides, turning once. Remove skillet from heat. Spread Dijon-Style Mustard on tops of chops; sprinkle with pecan mixture, lightly pressing into mustard.

3. Place skillet in oven. Bake for 3 to 4 minutes or until chops are done (145°F).

WALNUT-CRUSTED PORK WITH BLACKBERRY SPINACH SALAD

PREP: 30 minutes COOK: 4 minutes MAKES: 4 servings

PORK HAS A NATURALLY SWEET TASTE THAT PAIRS WELL WITH FRUIT. ALTHOUGH THE USUAL SUSPECTS ARE FALL FRUITS SUCH AS APPLES AND PEARS—OR STONE FRUITS SUCH AS PEACHES, PLUMS, AND APRICOTS—PORK IS ALSO DELICIOUS WITH BLACKBERRIES, WHICH HAVE A SWEET-TART, WINELIKE FLAVOR.

1⅔ cups blackberries
1 tablespoon plus 1½ teaspoons water
3 tablespoons walnut oil
1 tablespoon plus 1½ teaspoons white wine vinegar
2 eggs
¾ cup almond meal
⅓ cup finely chopped walnuts
1 tablespoon plus 1½ teaspoons Mediterranean Seasoning (see recipe)
4 pork cutlets or boneless pork loin chops (1 to 1½ pounds total)
6 cups fresh baby spinach leaves
½ cup torn fresh basil leaves
½ cup slivered red onion
½ cup chopped walnuts, toasted (see tip)
¼ cup refined coconut oil

1. For blackberry vinaigrette, in a small saucepan combine 1 cup of the blackberries and the water. Bring to boiling; reduce heat. Simmer, covered, for 4 to 5 minutes or just until berries are softened and color turns to a bright maroon, stirring occasionally. Remove from the heat; cool slightly. Pour undrained blackberries into a blender or

food processor; cover and blend or process until smooth. Using the back of a spoon, press pureed berries through a fine-mesh sieve; discard seeds and solids. In a medium bowl whisk together strained berries, walnut oil, and vinegar; set aside.

2. Line a large baking sheet with parchment paper; set aside. In a shallow dish lightly beat eggs well with a fork. In another shallow dish combine almond meal, the ⅓ cup finely chopped walnuts, and Mediterranean Seasoning. Dip pork cutlets, one at a time, in eggs and then in walnut mixture, turning to coat evenly. Place coated pork cutlets on a prepared baking sheet; set aside.

3. In a large bowl combine spinach and basil. Divide greens among four serving plates, arranging them along one side of the plates. Top with remaining ⅔ cup berries, the red onion, and the ½ cup toasted walnuts. Drizzle with blackberry vinaigrette.

4. In an extra-large skillet heat coconut oil over medium-high heat. Add pork cutlets to skillet; cook about 4 minutes or until done (145°F), turning once. Add pork cutlets to plates with salad.

PORK SCHNITZEL WITH SWEET-AND-SOUR RED CABBAGE

PREP: 20 minutes COOK: 45 minutes MAKES: 4 servings

IN THE "PALEO PRINCIPLES" SECTION OF THIS BOOK, ALMOND FLOUR (ALSO CALLED ALMOND MEAL) IS LISTED AS A NON-PALEO INGREDIENT—NOT BECAUSE ALMOND FLOUR IS INHERENTLY BAD, BUT BECAUSE IT IS FREQUENTLY USED TO CREATE ANALOGS OF WHEAT-FLOUR BROWNIES, CAKES, COOKIES, ETC., THAT SHOULD NOT BE A REGULAR PART OF A REAL PALEO DIET®. USED IN MODERATION AS COATING FOR A THIN SCALLOP OF PAN-FRIED PORK OR POULTRY, AS IT IS HERE, IS NOT A PROBLEM.

CABBAGE
- 2 tablespoons olive oil
- 1 cup chopped red onion
- 6 cups thinly sliced red cabbage (about ½ of a head)
- 2 Granny Smith apples, peeled, cored, and diced
- ¾ cup fresh orange juice
- 3 tablespoons cider vinegar
- ½ teaspoon caraway seeds
- ½ teaspoon celery seeds
- ½ teaspoon black pepper

PORK
- 4 boneless pork loin chops, cut ½ inch thick
- 2 cups almond flour
- 1 tablespoon dried lemon peel
- 2 teaspoons black pepper
- ¾ teaspoon ground allspice
- 1 large egg

¼ cup almond milk

3 tablespoons olive oil

Lemon wedges

1. For sweet-and-sour cabbage, in a 6-quart Dutch oven heat olive oil over medium-low heat. Add onion; cook for 6 to 8 minutes or until tender and lightly browned. Add cabbage; cook and stir for 6 to 8 minutes or until cabbage is crisp-tender. Add apples, orange juice, vinegar, caraway seeds, celery seeds, and ½ teaspoon pepper. Bring to boiling; reduce heat to low. Cover and cook for 30 minutes, stirring occasionally. Uncover and cook until liquid is reduced slightly.

2. Meanwhile, for pork, place chops between two sheets of plastic wrap or waxed paper. Using the flat side of a meat mallet or rolling pin, pound to about ¼ inch thickness; set aside.

3. In a shallow dish combine almond flour, dried lemon peel, 2 teaspoons pepper, and allspice. In another shallow dish whisk together the egg and almond milk. Lightly coat the pork cutlets in the seasoned flour, shaking off excess. Dip in the egg mixture, then again into the seasoned flour, shaking off excess. Repeat with remaining cutlets.

4. In a large skillet heat olive oil over medium-high heat. Add 2 cutlets to the pan. Cook for 6 to 8 minutes or until cutlets are golden brown and cooked through, turning once. Transfer cutlets to a warm platter. Repeat with remaining 2 cutlets.

5. Serve cutlets with cabbage and lemon wedges.

ROASTED TURKEY WITH GARLICKY MASHED ROOTS

PREP: 1 hour ROAST: 2 hours 45 minutes STAND: 15 minutes MAKES: 12 to 14 servings

LOOK FOR A TURKEY THAT HAS NOT BEEN INJECTED WITH A SALT SOLUTION. IF THE LABEL SAYS "ENHANCED" OR "SELF-BASTING," IT LIKELY IS FULL OF SODIUM AND OTHER ADDITIVES.

- 1 12- to 14-pound turkey
- 2 tablespoons Mediterranean Seasoning (see recipe)
- ¼ cup olive oil
- 3 pounds medium carrots, peeled, trimmed, and halved or quartered lengthwise
- 1 recipe Garlicky Mashed Roots (see recipe, below)

1. Preheat oven to 425°F. Remove neck and giblets from turkey; reserve for another use if desired. Carefully loosen skin from the edge of the breast. Run your fingers under the skin to create a pocket on top of the breast and on top of the drumsticks. Spoon 1 tablespoon of the Mediterranean Seasoning under the skin; use your fingers to evenly spread it over the breast and drumsticks. Pull neck skin to the back; fasten with a skewer. Tuck ends of drumsticks under the band of skin across the tail. If there is no band of skin, tie drumsticks securely to the tail with 100%-cotton kitchen string. Twist wing tips under the back.

2. Place turkey, breast side up, on a rack in a shallow extra-large roasting pan. Brush turkey with 2 tablespoons of the oil. Sprinkle turkey with remaining Mediterranean Seasoning. Insert an oven-going meat thermometer into

the center of an inside thigh muscle; the thermometer should not touch bone. Cover turkey loosely with foil.

3. Roast for 30 minutes. Reduce oven temperature to 325°F. Roast for 1½ hours. In an extra-large bowl combine carrots and the remaining 2 tablespoons oil; toss to coat. Spread carrots in a large rimmed baking pan. Remove foil from turkey and cut band of skin or string between drumsticks. Roast carrots and turkey for 45 minutes to 1¼ hours more or until the thermometer registers 175°F.

4. Remove turkey from oven. Cover; let stand for 15 to 20 minutes before carving. Serve turkey with carrots and Garlicky Mashed Roots.

Garlicky Mashed Roots: Trim and peel 3 to 3½ pounds rutabagas and 1½ to 2 pounds celery root; cut into 2-inch pieces. In a 6-quart pot cook rutabagas and celery root in enough boiling water to cover for 25 to 30 minutes or until very tender. Meanwhile, in a small saucepan combine 3 tablespoons extra virgin oil and 6 to 8 cloves minced garlic. Cook over low heat for 5 to 10 minutes or until garlic is very fragrant but not browned. Carefully add ¾ cup Chicken Bone Broth (see recipe) or no-salt-added chicken broth. Bring to boiling; remove from heat. Drain vegetables and return to the pot. Mash vegetables with a potato masher or beat with an electric mixer on low. Add ½ teaspoon black pepper. Gradually mash or beat in broth mixture until vegetables are combined and nearly smooth. If necessary, add an additional ¼ cup Chicken Bone Broth to make desired consistency.

STUFFED TURKEY BREAST WITH PESTO SAUCE AND ARUGULA SALAD

PREP: 30 minutes ROAST: 1 hour 30 minutes STAND: 20 minutes MAKES: 6 servings

THIS IS FOR THE WHITE-MEAT LOVERS OUT THERE—A CRISP-SKINNED BREAST OF TURKEY STUFFED WITH DRIED TOMATOES, BASIL, AND MEDITERRANEAN SPICES. LEFTOVERS MAKE A GREAT LUNCH.

- 1 cup unsulfured dried tomatoes (not oil-packed)
- 1 4-pound boneless turkey breast half with skin
- 3 teaspoons Mediterranean Seasoning (see recipe)
- 1 cup loosely packed fresh basil leaves
- 1 tablespoon olive oil
- 8 ounces baby arugula
- 3 large tomatoes, halved and sliced
- ¼ cup olive oil
- 2 tablespoons red wine vinegar
- Black pepper
- 1½ cups Basil Pesto (see recipe)

1. Preheat oven to 375°F. In a small bowl pour enough boiling water over dried tomatoes to cover. Let stand for 5 minutes; drain and finely chop.

2. Place turkey breast, skin side down, on a large sheet of plastic wrap. Place another sheet of plastic wrap over turkey. Using the flat side of a meat mallet, gently pound breast to an even thickness, about ¾ inch thick. Discard plastic wrap. Sprinkle 1½ teaspoons of the Mediterranean Seasoning over the meat. Top with the tomatoes and basil leaves. Carefully roll up turkey breast, keeping skin on the

outside. Using 100%-cotton kitchen string, tie roast in four to six places to secure. Brush with 1 tablespoon olive oil. Sprinkle roast with the remaining 1½ teaspoons Mediterranean Seasoning.

3. Place roast on a rack set in a shallow pan with the skin side up. Roast, uncovered, for 1½ hours or until an instant-read thermometer inserted near the center registers 165°F and skin is golden brown and crisp. Remove turkey from oven. Cover loosely with foil; let stand for 20 minutes before slicing.

4. For arugula salad, in a large bowl combine arugula, tomatoes, ¼ cup olive oil, the vinegar, and pepper to taste. Remove strings from roast. Thinly slice turkey. Serve with arugula salad and Basil Pesto.

SPICED TURKEY BREAST WITH CHERRY BBQ SAUCE

PREP: 15 minutes ROAST: 1 hour 15 minutes STAND: 45 minutes MAKES: 6 to 8 servings

THIS IS A NICE RECIPE FOR SERVING A CROWD AT A BACKYARD BARBECUE WHEN YOU WANT TO DO SOMETHING OTHER THAN BURGERS. SERVE IT WITH A CRISP SALAD, SUCH AS CRUNCHY BROCCOLI SALAD (SEE RECIPE) OR SHAVED BRUSSELS SPROUTS SALAD (SEE RECIPE).

1 4- to 5-pound whole bone-in turkey breast
3 tablespoons Smoky Seasoning (see recipe)
2 tablespoons fresh lemon juice
3 tablespoons olive oil
1 cup dry white wine, such as Sauvignon Blanc
1 cup fresh or frozen unsweetened Bing cherries, pitted and chopped
⅓ cup water
1 cup BBQ Sauce (see recipe)

1. Let turkey breast stand at room temperature for 30 minutes. Preheat oven to 325°F. Place the turkey breast, skin side up, on a rack in a roasting pan.

2. In a small bowl combine the Smoky Seasoning, lemon juice, and olive oil to make a paste. Loosen the skin from the meat; gently spread half of the paste onto the meat under the skin. Spread the remaining paste evenly over the skin. Pour the wine into the bottom of the roasting pan.

3. Roast for 1¼ to 1½ hours or until the skin is golden brown and an instant-read thermometer inserted into center of roast (not touching bone) registers 170°F, turning the

roasting pan halfway through cooking time. Let stand for 15 to 30 minutes before carving.

4. Meanwhile, for Cherry BBQ Sauce, in a medium saucepan combine cherries and the water. Bring to boiling; reduce heat. Simmer, uncovered, for 5 minutes. Stir in BBQ Sauce; simmer for 5 minutes. Serve warm or at room temperature with the turkey.

WINE-BRAISED TURKEY TENDERLOIN

PREP: 30 minutes COOK: 35 minutes MAKES: 4 servings

COOKING THE PAN-SEARED TURKEY IN A COMBINATION OF WINE, CHOPPED ROMA TOMATOES, CHICKEN BROTH, FRESH HERBS, AND CRUSHED RED PEPPER INFUSES IT WITH GREAT FLAVOR. SERVE THIS STEWLIKE DISH IN SHALLOW BOWLS AND WITH BIG SPOONS TO GET SOME OF THE TASTY BROTH WITH EVERY BITE.

2 8- to 12-ounce turkey tenderloins, cut into 1-inch pieces
2 tablespoons no-salt-added poultry seasoning
2 tablespoons olive oil
6 cloves garlic, minced (1 tablespoon)
1 cup chopped onion
½ cup chopped celery
6 roma tomatoes, seeded and chopped (about 3 cups)
½ cup dry white wine, such as Sauvignon Blanc
½ cup Chicken Bone Broth (see recipe) or no-salt-added chicken broth
½ teaspoon finely snipped fresh rosemary
¼ to ½ teaspoon crushed red pepper
½ cup fresh basil leaves, chopped
½ cup snipped fresh parsley

1. In a large bowl toss turkey pieces with poultry seasoning to coat. In an extra-large nonstick skillet heat 1 tablespoon of the olive oil over medium heat. Cook turkey in batches in hot oil until browned on all sides. (Turkey does not need to be cooked through.) Transfer to a plate and keep warm.

2. Add the remaining 1 tablespoon olive oil to the pan. Increase heat to medium-high. Add the garlic; cook and stir for 1 minute. Add onion and celery; cook and stir for 5

minutes. Add the turkey and any juices from the plate, tomatoes, wine, Chicken Bone Broth, rosemary, and crushed red pepper. Reduce heat to medium-low. Cover and cook for 20 minutes, stirring occasionally. Add basil and parsley. Uncover and cook for 5 minutes more or until turkey is no longer pink.

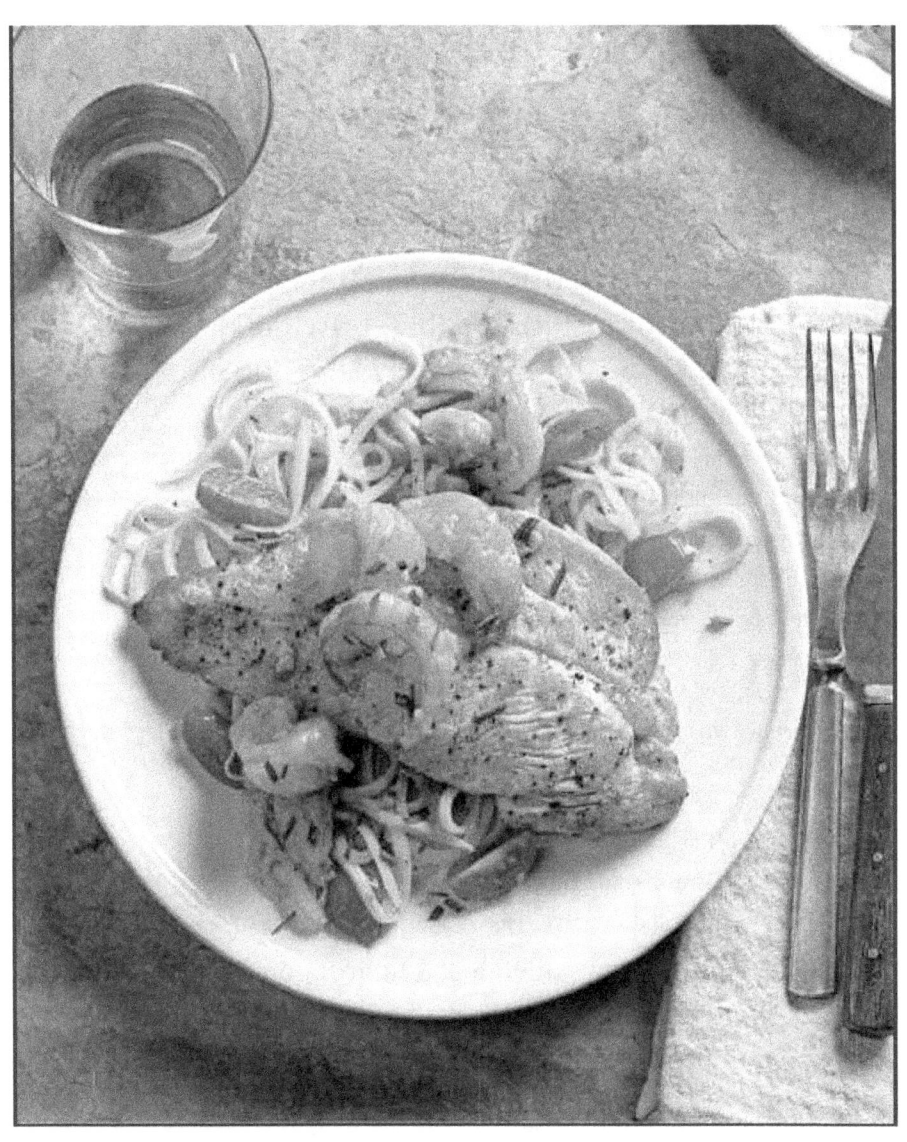

PAN-SAUTÉED TURKEY BREAST WITH CHIVE SCAMPI SAUCE

PREP: 30 minutes COOK: 15 minutes MAKES: 4 servings PHOTO

TO CUT THE TURKEY TENDERLOINS IN HALF HORIZONTALLY AS EVENLY AS POSSIBLE, LIGHTLY PRESS DOWN ON EACH ONE WITH THE PALM OF YOUR HAND, APPLYING CONSISTENT PRESSURE, AS YOU CUT THROUGH THE MEAT.

¼ cup olive oil

2 8- to 12-ounce turkey breast tenderloins, cut in half horizontally

¼ teaspoon freshly ground black pepper

3 tablespoons olive oil

4 cloves garlic, minced

8 ounces peeled and deveined medium shrimp, tails removed and halved lengthwise

¼ cup dry white wine, Chicken Bone Broth (see recipe), or no-salt-added chicken broth

2 tablespoons snipped fresh chives

½ teaspoon finely shredded lemon peel

1 tablespoon fresh lemon juice

Squash Noodles and Tomatoes (see recipe, below) (optional)

1. In an extra-large skillet heat 1 tablespoon of the olive oil over medium-high heat. Add turkey to skillet; sprinkle with pepper. Reduce heat to medium. Cook for 12 to 15 minutes or until no longer pink and juices run clear (165°F), turning once halfway through cooking time. Remove turkey steaks from skillet. Cover with foil to keep warm.

2. For sauce, in the same skillet heat the 3 tablespoons oil over medium heat. Add garlic; cook for 30 seconds. Stir in

shrimp; cook and stir for 1 minute. Stir in wine, chives, and lemon peel; cook and stir for 1 minute more or until shrimp are opaque. Remove from heat; stir in lemon juice. To serve, spoon sauce over turkey steaks. If desired, serve with Squash Noodles and Tomatoes.

Squash Noodles and Tomatoes: Using a mandoline or julienne peeler, slice 2 yellow summer squash into julienne strips. In a large skillet heat 1 tablespoon extra virgin olive oil over medium-high heat. Add squash strips; cook for 2 minutes. Add 1 cup quartered grape tomatoes and ¼ teaspoon freshly ground black pepper; cook for 2 minutes more or until squash is crisp-tender.

BRAISED TURKEY LEGS WITH ROOT VEGETABLES

PREP: 30 minutes COOK: 1 hour 45 minutes MAKES: 4 servings

THIS IS ONE OF THOSE DISHES YOU WANT TO MAKE ON A CRISP FALL AFTERNOON WHEN YOU HAVE TIME TO TAKE A WALK WHILE IT SIMMERS IN THE OVEN. IF THE EXERCISE DOESN'T STIR UP AN APPETITE, THE WONDERFUL AROMA WHEN YOU WALK THROUGH THE DOOR CERTAINLY WILL.

- 3 tablespoons olive oil
- 4 20- to 24-ounce turkey legs
- ½ teaspoon freshly ground black pepper
- 6 cloves garlic, peeled and crushed
- 1½ teaspoons fennel seeds, bruised
- 1 teaspoon whole allspice, bruised*
- 1½ cups Chicken Bone Broth (see recipe) or no-salt-added chicken broth
- 2 sprigs fresh rosemary
- 2 sprigs fresh thyme
- 1 bay leaf
- 2 large onions, peeled and cut into 8 wedges each
- 6 large carrots, peeled and cut into 1-inch slices
- 2 large turnips, peeled and cut into 1-inch cubes
- 2 medium parsnips, peeled and cut into 1-inch slices**
- 1 celery root, peeled and cut into 1-inch pieces

1. Preheat oven to 350°F. In a large skillet heat the olive oil over medium-high heat until shimmering. Add 2 of the turkey legs. Cook about 8 minutes or until legs are golden brown and crisp on all sides, turning to brown evenly. Transfer turkey legs to a plate; repeat with remaining 2 turkey legs. Set aside.

2. Add pepper, garlic, fennel seeds, and allspice seeds to the skillet. Cook and stir over medium heat for 1 to 2 minutes or until fragrant. Stir in Chicken Bone Broth, rosemary, thyme, and bay leaf. Bring to boiling, stirring to scrape browned bits from the bottom of the skillet. Remove skillet from heat and set aside.

3. In an extra-large Dutch oven with a tight-fitting lid combine onions, carrots, turnips, parsnips, and celery root. Add liquid from skillet; toss to coat. Press turkey legs into the vegetable mixture. Cover with lid.

4. Bake about 1 hour 45 minutes or until vegetables are tender and turkey is cooked through. Serve turkey legs and vegetables in large shallow bowls. Drizzle juices from pan over top.

*Tip: To bruise allspice and fennel seeds, place seeds on a cutting board. Using a flat side of a chef's knife, press down to lightly crush the seeds.

**Tip: Cube any large pieces from the tops of the parsnips.

HERBED TURKEY MEAT LOAF WITH CARAMELIZED ONION KETCHUP AND ROASTED CABBAGE WEDGES

PREP: 15 minutes COOK: 30 minutes BAKE: 1 hour 10 minutes STAND: 5 minutes MAKES: 4 servings

CLASSIC KETCHUP-TOPPED MEAT LOAF IS DEFINITELY ON THE PALEO MENU WHEN THE KETCHUP (SEE RECIPE) IS FREE OF SALT AND ADDED SUGARS. HERE THE KETCHUP IS STIRRED TOGETHER WITH CARAMELIZED ONIONS, WHICH ARE PILED ON TOP OF THE MEAT LOAF BEFORE BAKING.

1½ pounds ground turkey

2 eggs, lightly beaten

½ cup almond meal

⅓ cup snipped fresh parsley

¼ cup thinly sliced scallions (2)

1 tablespoon snipped fresh sage or 1 teaspoon dried sage, crushed

1 tablespoon snipped fresh thyme or 1 teaspoon dried thyme, crushed

¼ teaspoon black pepper

2 tablespoons olive oil

2 sweet onions, halved and thinly sliced

1 cup Paleo Ketchup (see recipe)

1 small head cabbage, halved, cored, and cut into 8 wedges

½ to 1 teaspoon crushed red pepper

1. Preheat oven to 350°F. Line a large roasting pan with parchment paper; set aside. In a large bowl combine ground turkey, eggs, almond meal, parsley, scallions, sage, thyme, and black pepper. In the prepared roasting pan shape turkey mixture into an 8×4-inch loaf. Bake for 30 minutes.

2. Meanwhile, for the caramelized onion ketchup, in a large skillet heat 1 tablespoon of the olive oil over medium heat. Add onions; cook about 5 minutes or until onions just start to brown, stirring frequently. Reduce heat to medium-low; cook about 25 minutes or until golden and very soft, stirring occasionally. Remove from heat; stir in Paleo Ketchup.

3. Spoon some of the caramelized onion ketchup over turkey loaf. Arrange cabbage wedges around loaf. Drizzle cabbage with the remaining 1 tablespoon olive oil; sprinkle with crushed red pepper. Bake about 40 minutes or until an instant-read thermometer inserted in center of loaf registers 165°F, topping with additional caramelized onion ketchup and turning the cabbage wedges after 20 minutes. Let turkey loaf stand for 5 to 10 minutes before slicing.

4. Serve turkey loaf with cabbage wedges and any remaining caramelized onion ketchup.

TURKEY POSOLE

PREP: 20 minutes BROIL: 8 minutes COOK: 16 minutes MAKES: 4 servings

THE TOPPINGS ON THIS WARMING, MEXICAN-STYLE SOUP ARE MORE THAN GARNISHES. THE CILANTRO ADDS DISTINCTIVE FLAVOR, AVOCADO CONTRIBUTES CREAMINESS—AND TOASTED PEPITAS PROVIDE A DELIGHTFUL CRUNCH.

8 fresh tomatillos
1¼ to 1½ pounds ground turkey
1 red sweet pepper, seeded and cut into thin bite-size strips
½ cup chopped onion (1 medium)
6 cloves garlic, minced (1 tablespoon)
1 tablespoon Mexican Seasoning (see recipe)
2 cups Chicken Bone Broth (see recipe) or no-salt-added chicken broth
1 14.5-ounce can no-salt-added fire-roasted tomatoes, undrained
1 jalapeño or serrano chile pepper, seeded and minced (see tip)
1 medium avocado, halved, peeled, seeded, and thinly sliced
¼ cup unsalted pepitas, toasted (see tip)
¼ cup snipped fresh cilantro
Lime wedges

1. Preheat the broiler. Remove husks from tomatillos and discard. Wash tomatillos and cut into halves. Place tomatillo halves on the unheated rack of a broiler pan. Broil 4 to 5 inches from the heat for 8 to 10 minutes or until lightly charred, turning once halfway through broiling. Cool slightly on pan on a wire rack.

2. Meanwhile, in a large skillet cook turkey, sweet pepper, and onion over medium-high heat for 5 to 10 minutes or until turkey is browned and vegetables are tender, stirring with a wooden spoon to break up meat as it cooks. Drain off fat

if necessary. Add garlic and Mexican Seasoning. Cook and stir for 1 minute more.

3. In a blender combine about two-thirds of the charred tomatillos and 1 cup of the Chicken Bone Broth. Cover and blend until smooth. Add to turkey mixture in skillet. Stir in the remaining 1 cup Chicken Bone Broth, undrained tomatoes, and chile pepper. Coarsely chop the remaining tomatillos; add to the turkey mixture. Bring to boiling; reduce heat. Cover and simmer for 10 minutes.

4. To serve, ladle soup into shallow serving bowls. Top with avocado, pepitas, and cilantro. Pass lime wedges to squeeze over soup.

CHICKEN BONE BROTH

PREP: 15 minutes ROAST: 30 minutes COOK: 4 hours CHILL: overnight MAKES: about 10 cups

FOR THE FRESHEST, BEST TASTE—AND HIGHEST NUTRIENT CONTENT—USE HOMEMADE CHICKEN BROTH IN YOUR RECIPES. (IT ALSO DOESN'T CONTAIN ANY SALT, PRESERVATIVES, OR ADDITIVES.) ROASTING THE BONES BEFORE SIMMERING ENHANCES FLAVOR. AS THEY SLOWLY COOK IN LIQUID, THE BONES INFUSE THE BROTH WITH MINERALS SUCH AS CALCIUM, PHOSPHORUS, MAGNESIUM, AND POTASSIUM. THE SLOW COOKER VARIATION BELOW MAKES IT ESPECIALLY EASY TO DO. FREEZE IT IN 2- AND 4-CUP CONTAINERS AND THAW ONLY WHAT YOU NEED.

- 2 pounds chicken wings and backs
- 4 carrots, chopped
- 2 large leeks, white and pale green parts only, thinly sliced
- 2 stalks celery with leaves, coarsely chopped
- 1 parsnip, coarsely chopped
- 6 large sprigs Italian (flat-leaf) parsley
- 6 sprigs fresh thyme
- 4 cloves garlic, halved
- 2 teaspoons whole black peppercorns
- 2 whole cloves
- Cold water

1. Preheat oven to 425°F. Arrange chicken wings and backs on a large baking sheet; roast for 30 to 35 minutes or until well browned.

2. Transfer browned chicken pieces and any browned bits accumulated on the baking sheet to a large stockpot. Add

carrots, leeks, celery, parsnip, parsley, thyme, garlic, peppercorns, and cloves. Add enough cold water (about 12 cups) to a large stockpot to cover chicken and vegetables. Bring to simmering over medium heat; adjust heat to maintain broth at a very low simmer, with bubbles just breaking the surface. Cover and simmer for 4 hours.

3. Strain hot broth through a large colander lined with two layers of damp 100%-cotton cheesecloth. Discard solids. Cover broth and chill overnight. Before using, remove fat layer from top of broth and discard.

Tip: To clarify stock (optional), in a small bowl combine 1 egg white, 1 crushed eggshell, and ¼ cup cold water. Stir mixture into strained stock in pot. Return to boiling. Remove from heat; let stand for 5 minutes. Strain hot broth through a colander lined with a fresh double layer of 100%-cotton cheesecloth. Chill and skim fat before using.

Slow Cooker Directions: Prepare as directed, except in Step 2 place ingredients in a 5- to 6-quart slow cooker. Cover and cook on low-heat setting for 12 to 14 hours. Continue as directed in Step 3. Makes about 10 cups.

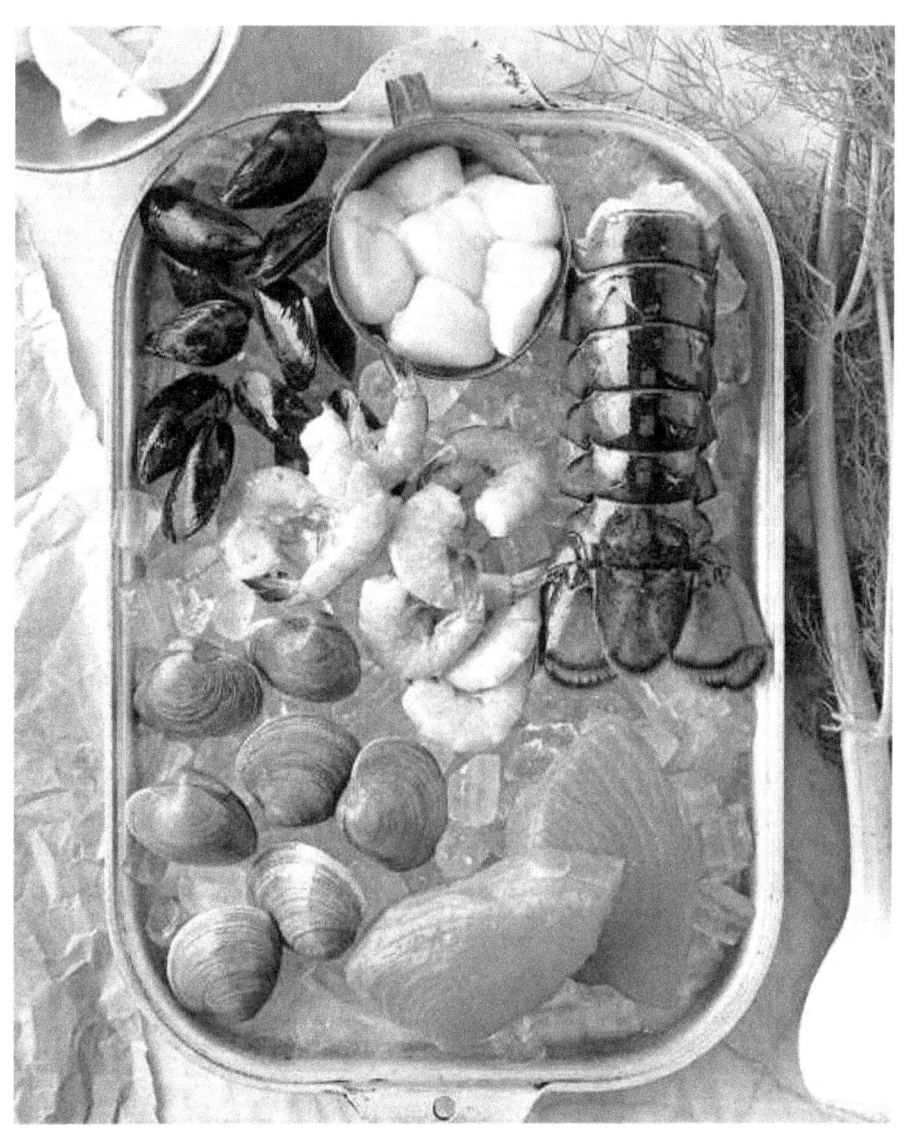

GREEN HARISSA SALMON

PREP: 25 minutes BAKE: 10 minutes GRILL: 8 minutes MAKES: 4 servings PHOTO

A STANDARD VEGETABLE PEELER IS USED TO SHAVE FRESH RAW ASPARAGUS INTO THIN RIBBONS FOR THE SALAD. TOSSED WITH BRIGHT CITRUS VINAIGRETTE (SEE RECIPE) AND TOPPED WITH SMOKY TOASTED SUNFLOWER SEEDS, IT'S A REFRESHING ACCOMPANIMENT TO THE SALMON AND SPICY GREEN HERB SAUCE.

SALMON
4 6- to 8-ounce fresh or frozen skinless salmon fillets, about 1 inch thick
Olive oil

HARISSA
1½ teaspoons cumin seeds
1½ teaspoons coriander seeds
1 cup tightly packed fresh parsley leaves
1 cup roughly chopped fresh cilantro (leaves and stems)
2 jalapeños, seeded and coarsely chopped (see tip)
1 scallion, cut up
2 cloves garlic
1 teaspoon finely shredded lemon peel
2 tablespoons fresh lemon juice
⅓ cup olive oil

SPICED SUNFLOWER SEEDS
⅓ cup raw sunflower seeds
1 teaspoon olive oil
1 teaspoon Smoky Seasoning (see recipe)

SALAD
12 large asparagus spears, trimmed (about 1 pound)
⅓ cup Bright Citrus Vinaigrette (see recipe)

1. Thaw fish, if frozen; pat dry with paper towels. Brush both sides of fish lightly with olive oil. Set aside.

2. For harissa, in a small skillet toast cumin seeds and coriander seeds over medium-low heat for 3 to 4 minutes or until lightly toasted and fragrant. In a food processor combine toasted cumin and coriander seeds, the parsley, cilantro, jalapeños, scallion, garlic, lemon peel, lemon juice, and olive oil. Process until smooth. Set aside.

3. For spiced sunflower seeds, preheat oven to 300°F. Line a baking sheet with parchment paper; set aside. In a small bowl combine sunflower seeds and 1 teaspoon olive oil. Sprinkle the Smoky Seasoning over the seeds; stir to coat. Spread sunflower seeds evenly on the parchment paper. Bake about 10 minutes or until lightly toasted.

4. For a charcoal or gas grill, place salmon on a greased grill rack directly over medium heat. Cover and grill for 8 to 12 minutes or until fish begins to flake when tested with a fork, turning once halfway through grilling.

5. Meanwhile, for salad, using a vegetable peeler, shave asparagus spears into long thin ribbons. Transfer to a platter or medium bowl. (The tips will snap off as the spears get thinner; add them to platter or bowl.) Drizzle the Bright Citrus Vinaigrette over shaved spears. Sprinkle with spiced sunflower seeds.

6. To serve, place a fillet on each of four plates; spoon some of the green harissa on each fillet. Serve with shaved asparagus salad.

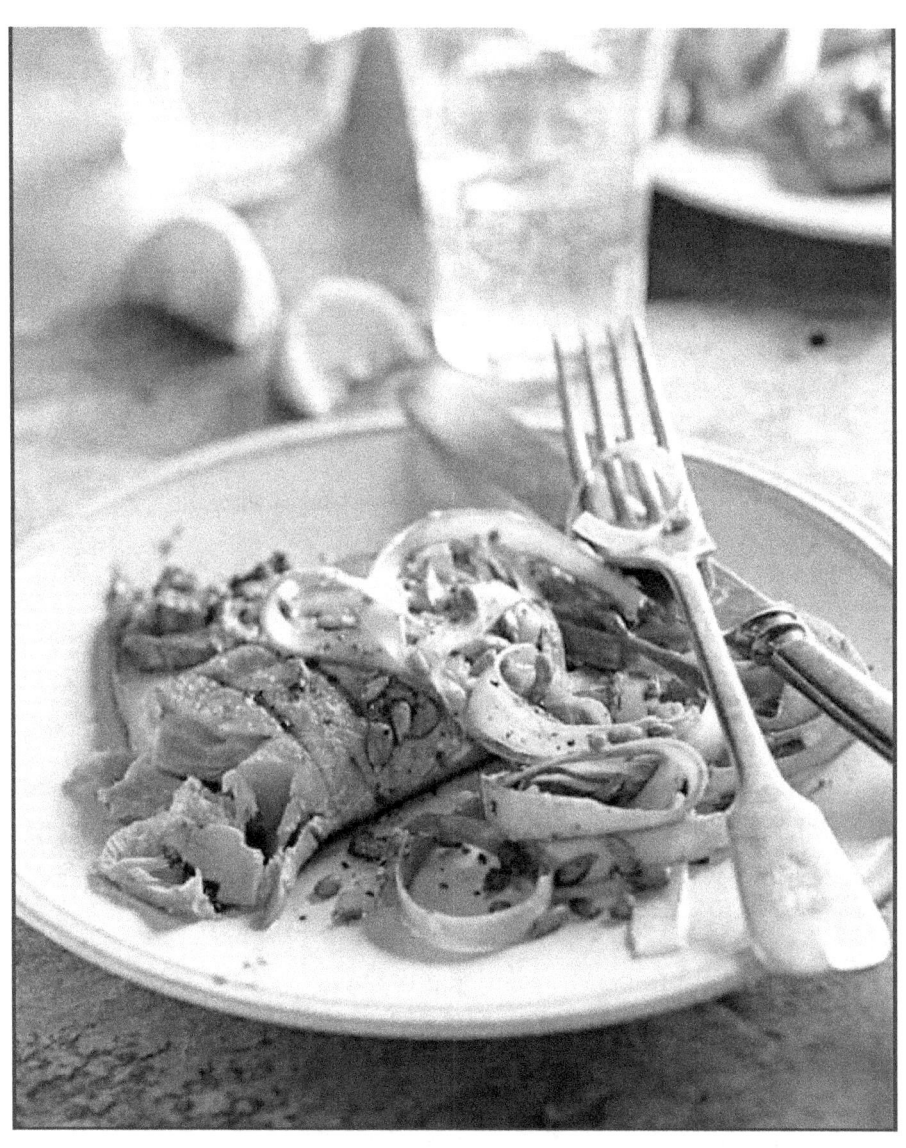

GRILLED SALMON WITH MARINATED ARTICHOKE HEART SALAD

PREP: 20 minutes GRILL: 12 minutes MAKES: 4 servings

OFTENTIMES, THE BEST TOOLS FOR TOSSING A SALAD ARE YOUR HANDS. GETTING THE TENDER LETTUCES AND GRILLED ARTICHOKES TO INCORPORATE EVENLY IN THIS SALAD IS BEST DONE WITH CLEAN HANDS.

4 6-ounce fresh or frozen salmon fillets
1 9-ounce package frozen artichoke hearts, thawed and drained
5 tablespoons olive oil
2 tablespoons minced shallots
1 tablespoon finely shredded lemon peel
¼ cup fresh lemon juice
3 tablespoons snipped fresh oregano
½ teaspoon freshly ground black pepper
1 tablespoon Mediterranean Seasoning (see recipe)
1 5-ounce package mixed baby lettuces

1. Thaw fish, if frozen. Rinse fish; pat dry with paper towels. Set fish aside.

2. In a medium bowl toss artichoke hearts with 2 tablespoons of the olive oil; set aside. In a large bowl combine 2 tablespoons of the olive oil, the shallots, lemon peel, lemon juice, and oregano; set aside.

3. For a charcoal or gas grill, place the artichoke hearts in a grill basket and grill directly over medium-high heat. Cover and grill for 6 to 8 minutes or until nicely charred and heated through, stirring frequently. Remove artichokes from grill. Let cool 5 minutes, then add

artichokes to shallot mixture. Season with pepper; toss to coat. Set aside.

4. Brush salmon with the remaining 1 tablespoon olive oil; sprinkle with the Mediterranean Seasoning. Place salmon on the grill rack, seasoned sides down, directly over medium-high heat. Cover and grill for 6 to 8 minutes or until fish begins to flake when tested with a fork, carefully turning once halfway through grilling.

5. Add lettuces to bowl with marinated artichokes; toss gently to coat. Serve salad with grilled salmon.

FLASH-ROASTED CHILE-SAGE SALMON WITH GREEN TOMATO SALSA

PREP: 35 minutes CHILL: 2 to 4 hours ROAST: 10 minutes MAKES: 4 servings

"FLASH-ROASTING" REFERS TO THE TECHNIQUE OF HEATING A DRY SKILLET IN THE OVEN AT A HIGH TEMPERATURE, ADDING SOME OIL AND THE FISH, CHICKEN, OR MEAT (IT SIZZLES!), THEN FINISHING THE DISH IN THE OVEN. FLASH-ROASTING CUTS DOWN ON COOKING TIME AND CREATES A DELICIOUSLY CRISP CRUST ON THE EXTERIOR—AND A JUICY, FLAVORFUL INTERIOR.

SALMON

- 4 5- to 6-ounce fresh or frozen salmon fillets
- 3 tablespoons olive oil
- ¼ cup finely chopped onion
- 2 cloves garlic, peeled and sliced
- 1 tablespoon ground coriander
- 1 teaspoon ground cumin
- 2 teaspoons sweet paprika
- 1 teaspoon dried oregano, crushed
- ¼ teaspoon cayenne pepper
- ⅓ cup fresh lime juice
- 1 tablespoon snipped fresh sage

GREEN TOMATO SALSA

- 1½ cups diced firm green tomatoes
- ⅓ cup finely chopped red onion
- 2 tablespoons snipped fresh cilantro
- 1 jalapeño, seeded and minced (see tip)
- 1 clove garlic, minced
- ½ teaspoon ground cumin

¼ teaspoon chili powder

2 to 3 tablespoons fresh lime juice

1. Thaw fish, if frozen. Rinse fish; pat dry with paper towels. Set fish aside.

2. For chile-sage paste, in a small saucepan combine 1 tablespoon of the olive oil, onion, and garlic. Cook over low heat for 1 to 2 minutes or until fragrant. Stir in coriander and cumin; cook and stir for 1 minute. Stir in paprika, oregano, and cayenne pepper; cook and stir for 1 minute. Add lime juice and sage; cook and stir about 3 minutes or just until a smooth paste forms; cool.

3. Using your fingers, coat both sides of fillets with chile-sage paste. Place fish in a glass or nonreactive dish; cover tightly with plastic wrap. Refrigerate for 2 to 4 hours.

4. Meanwhile, for salsa, in a medium bowl combine tomatoes, onion, cilantro, jalapeño, garlic, cumin, and chili powder. Toss well to mix. Drizzle with lime juice; toss to coat.

4. Using a rubber spatula, scrape as much paste as you can off of the salmon. Discard paste.

5. Place an extra-large cast-iron skillet in the oven. Turn oven to 500°F. Preheat oven with skillet in it.

6. Remove hot skillet from oven. Pour 1 tablespoon olive oil into the pan. Tip pan to cover the bottom of the skillet with oil. Place fillets in the skillet, skin sides down. Brush tops of fillets with the remaining 1 tablespoon olive oil.

7. Roast salmon about 10 minutes or until fish begins to flake when tested with a fork. Serve fish with salsa.

ROASTED SALMON AND ASPARAGUS EN PAPILLOTE WITH LEMON-HAZELNUT PESTO

PREP: 20 minutes ROAST: 17 minutes MAKES: 4 servings

COOKING "EN PAPILLOTE" SIMPLY MEANS COOKING IN PAPER. IT IS A BEAUTIFUL WAY TO COOK FOR MANY REASONS. THE FISH AND VEGETABLES STEAM INSIDE THE PARCHMENT PACKET, SEALING IN JUICES, FLAVOR, AND NUTRIENTS—AND THERE ARE NO POTS AND PANS TO WASH AFTERWARDS.

4 6-ounce fresh or frozen salmon fillets
1 cup lightly packed fresh basil leaves
1 cup lightly packed fresh parsley leaves
½ cup hazelnuts, toasted*
5 tablespoons olive oil
1 teaspoon finely shredded lemon peel
2 tablespoons fresh lemon juice
1 clove garlic, chopped
1 pound slender asparagus, trimmed
4 tablespoons dry white wine

1. Thaw salmon, if frozen. Rinse fish; pat dry with paper towels. Preheat oven to 400°F.

2. For pesto, in a blender or food processor combine basil, parsley, hazelnuts, olive oil, lemon peel, lemon juice, and garlic. Cover and blend or process until smooth; set aside.

3. Cut four 12-inch squares of parchment paper. For each packet, place a salmon fillet in the center of a parchment square. Top with one-fourth of the asparagus and 2 to 3

tablespoons pesto; drizzle with 1 tablespoon wine. Bring up two opposite sides of the parchment paper and fold together several times over fish. Fold ends of parchment to seal. Repeat to make three more packets.

4. Roast for 17 to 19 minutes or until fish begins to flake when tested with a fork (carefully open packet to check doneness).

*Tip: To toast hazelnuts, preheat oven to 350°F. Spread nuts in a single layer in a shallow baking pan. Bake for 8 to 10 minutes or until lightly toasted, stirring once to toast evenly. Cool nuts slightly. Place warm nuts on a clean kitchen towel; rub with the towel to remove the loose skins.

SPICE-RUBBED SALMON WITH MUSHROOM-APPLE PAN SAUCE

START TO FINISH: 40 minutes MAKES: 4 servings

THIS WHOLE SALMON FILLET TOPPED WITH A MIXTURE OF SAUTÉED MUSHROOMS, SHALLOT, RED-SKINNED APPLE SLICES—AND SERVED ON A BED OF BRIGHT-GREEN SPINACH—MAKES AN IMPRESSIVE DISH TO SERVE TO GUESTS.

1 1½-pound fresh or frozen whole salmon fillet, skin on
1 teaspoon fennel seeds, finely crushed*
½ teaspoon dried sage, crushed
½ teaspoon ground coriander
¼ teaspoon dry mustard
¼ teaspoon black pepper
2 tablespoons olive oil
1½ cups fresh cremini mushrooms, quartered
1 medium shallot, very thinly sliced
1 small cooking apple, quartered, cored, and thinly sliced
¼ cup dry white wine
4 cups fresh spinach
Small sprigs fresh sage (optional)

1. Thaw salmon, if frozen. Preheat oven to 425°F. Line a large baking sheet with parchment paper; set aside. Rinse fish; pat dry with paper towels. Place salmon, skin side down, on prepared baking sheet. In a small bowl combine fennel seeds, ½ teaspoon dried sage, coriander, mustard, and pepper. Sprinkle evenly over salmon; rub in with your fingers.

2. Measure thickness of fish. Roast salmon for 4 to 6 minutes per ½-inch thickness or until fish begins to flake when tested with a fork.

3. Meanwhile, for pan sauce, in a large skillet heat olive oil over medium heat. Add mushrooms and shallot; cook for 6 to 8 minutes or until mushrooms are tender and starting to brown, stirring occasionally. Add apple; cover and cook and stir for 4 minutes more. Carefully add wine. Cook, uncovered, for 2 to 3 minutes or until apple slices are just tender. Using a slotted spoon, transfer mushroom mixture to a medium bowl; cover to keep warm.

4. In the same skillet cook spinach for 1 minute or until spinach is just wilted, stirring constantly. Divide spinach among four serving plates. Cut salmon fillet into four equal portions, cutting to, but not through, the skin. Use a large spatula to lift salmon portions off of the skin; place one salmon portion on spinach on each plate. Spoon mushroom mixture evenly over salmon. If desired, garnish with fresh sage.

*Tip: Use a mortar and pestle or spice grinder to finely crush the fennel seeds.

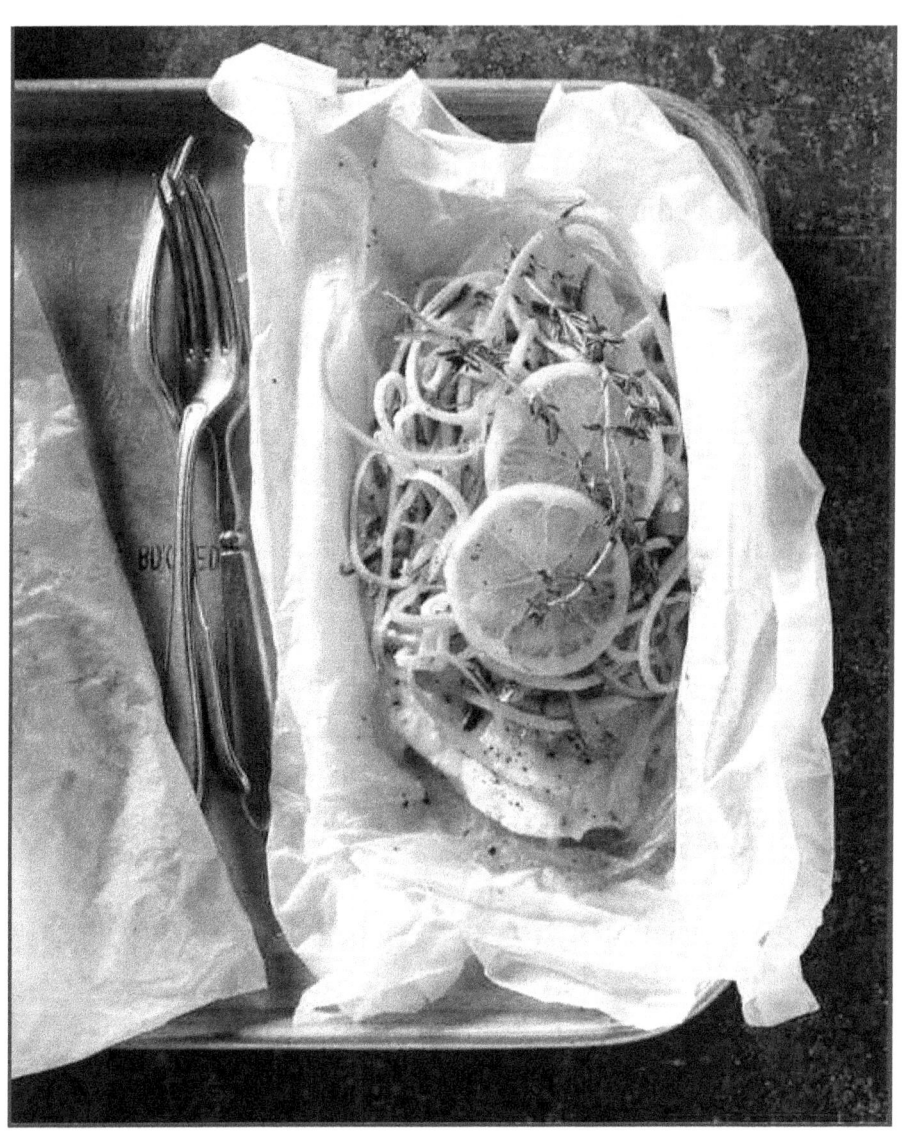

SOLE EN PAPILLOTE WITH JULIENNE VEGETABLES

PREP: 30 minutes BAKE: 12 minutes MAKES: 4 servings PHOTO

YOU CAN CERTAINLY JULIENNE VEGETABLES WITH A GOOD SHARP CHEF'S KNIFE, BUT IT IS VERY TIME-CONSUMING. A JULIENNE PEELER (SEE "EQUIPMENT") MAKES QUICK WORK OF CREATING LONG, THIN, CONSISTENTLY SHAPED STRIPS OF VEGETABLES.

4 6-ounce fresh or frozen sole, flounder, or other firm white fish fillets
1 zucchini, julienne cut
1 large carrot, julienne cut
½ of a red onion, julienne cut
2 roma tomatoes, seeded and finely chopped
2 cloves garlic, minced
1 tablespoon olive oil
½ teaspoon black pepper
1 lemon, cut into 8 thin slices, seeds removed
8 sprigs fresh thyme
4 teaspoons olive oil
¼ cup dry white wine

1. Thaw fish, if frozen. Preheat oven to 375°F. In a large bowl combine zucchini, carrot, onion, tomatoes, and garlic. Add 1 tablespoon olive oil and ¼ teaspoon of the pepper; toss well to combine. Set vegetables aside.

2. Cut four 14-inch squares of parchment paper. Rinse fish; pat dry with paper towels. Place a fillet in the center of each square. Sprinkle with the remaining ¼ teaspoon pepper. Arrange vegetables, lemon slices, and thyme sprigs on top

of fillets, dividing evenly. Drizzle each stack with 1 teaspoon olive oil and 1 tablespoon white wine.

3. Working with one packet at a time, bring up two opposite sides of the parchment paper and fold together several times over fish. Fold ends of parchment to seal.

4. Arrange packets on a large baking sheet. Bake about 12 minutes or until fish begins to flake when tested with a fork (carefully open packet to check doneness).

5. To serve, place each packet on a dinner plate; carefully open packets.

ARUGULA PESTO FISH TACOS WITH SMOKY LIME CREAM

PREP: 30 minutes GRILL: 4 to 6 minutes per ½-inch thickness MAKES: 6 servings

YOU CAN SUBSTITUTE COD FOR THE SOLE—JUST NOT TILAPIA. TILAPIA IS UNFORTUNATELY ONE OF THE WORST CHOICES FOR FISH. IT IS ALMOST UNIVERSALLY FARM-RAISED AND FREQUENTLY UNDER HORRIBLE CONDITIONS—SO WHILE TILAPIA IS NEARLY UBIQUITOUS, IT SHOULD BE AVOIDED.

- 4 4- to 5-ounce fresh or frozen sole fillets, about ½ inch thick
- 1 recipe Arugula Pesto (see recipe)
- ½ cup Cashew Cream (see recipe)
- 1 teaspoon Smoky Seasoning (see recipe)
- ½ teaspoon finely shredded lime peel
- 12 butterhead lettuce leaves
- 1 ripe avocado, halved, seeded, peeled, and cut into thin slices
- 1 cup chopped tomato
- ¼ cup snipped fresh cilantro
- 1 lime, cut into wedges

1. Thaw fish, if frozen. Rinse fish; pat dry with paper towels. Set fish aside.

2. Rub some of the Arugula Pesto on both sides of the fish.

3. For a charcoal or gas grill, place fish on a greased rack directly over medium heat. Cover and grill for 4 to 6 minutes or until fish begins to flake when tested with a fork, turning once halfway through grilling.

4. Meanwhile, for Smoky Lime Cream, in a small bowl stir together the Cashew Cream, Smoky Seasoning, and lime peel.

5. Using a fork, break fish into pieces. Fill butterhead leaves with fish, avocado slices, and tomato; sprinkle with cilantro. Drizzle tacos with Smoky Lime Cream. Serve with lime wedges to squeeze over tacos.

ALMOND-CRUSTED SOLE

PREP: 15 minutes COOK: 3 minutes MAKES: 2 servings

JUST A LITTLE BIT OF ALMOND FLOUR CREATES A NICE CRUST ON THIS EXTREMELY QUICK-COOKING PAN-FRIED FISH SERVED WITH CREAMY DILLED MAYONNAISE AND A SQUEEZE OF FRESH LEMON.

12 ounces fresh or frozen sole fillets
1 tablespoon Lemon-Herb Seasoning (see recipe)
¼ to ½ teaspoon black pepper
⅓ cup almond flour
2 to 3 tablespoons olive oil
¼ cup Paleo Mayo (see recipe)
1 teaspoon snipped fresh dill
Lemon wedges

1. Thaw fish, if frozen. Rinse fish; pat dry with paper towels. In a small bowl stir together the Lemon-Herb Seasoning and pepper. Coat both sides of fillets with seasoning mixture, pressing lightly to adhere. Spread almond flour on a large plate. Dredge one side of each fillet in the almond flour, pressing lightly to adhere.

2. In a large skillet heat enough oil to coat pan over medium-high heat. Add fish, coated sides down. Cook for 2 minutes. Carefully turn fish over; cook about 1 minute more or until the fish begins to flake when tested with a fork.

3. For sauce, in a small bowl stir together the Paleo Mayo and dill. Serve fish with sauce and lemon wedges.

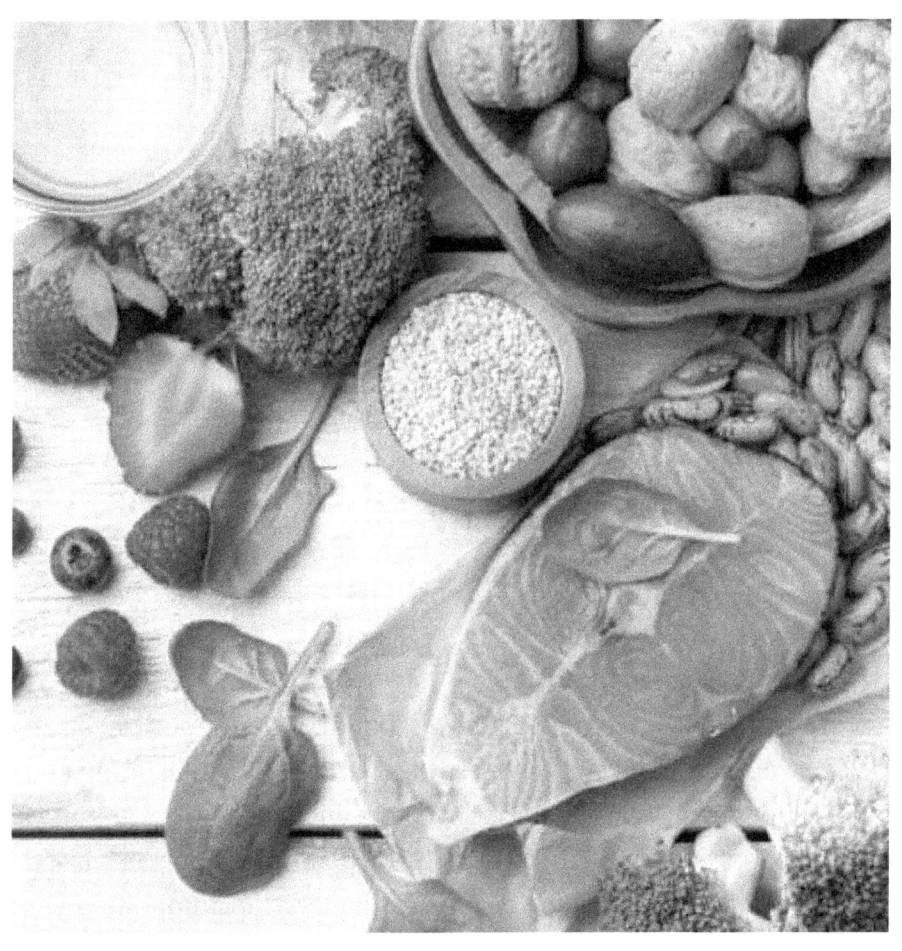

GRILLED COD AND ZUCCHINI PACKETS WITH SPICY MANGO-BASIL SAUCE

PREP: 20 minutes GRILL: 6 minutes MAKES: 4 servings

1 to 1½ pounds fresh or frozen cod, ½ to 1 inch thick
4 24-inch-long pieces 12-inch-wide foil
1 medium zucchini, cut into julienne strips
Lemon-Herb Seasoning (see recipe)
¼ cup Chipotle Paleo Mayo (see recipe)
1 to 2 tablespoons pureed ripe mango*
1 tablespoon fresh lime or lemon juice or rice wine vinegar
2 tablespoons snipped fresh basil

1. Thaw fish, if frozen. Rinse fish; pat dry with paper towels. Cut fish into four serving-size pieces.

2. Fold each piece of foil in half to create a double-thickness 12-inch square. Place one portion of fish in the middle of a foil square. Top with one-fourth of the zucchini. Sprinkle with Lemon-Herb Seasoning. Bring up two opposite sides of foil and fold several times over zucchini and fish. Fold ends of foil. Repeat to make three more packets. For sauce, in a small bowl stir together Chipotle Paleo Mayo, mango, lime juice, and basil; set aside.

3. For a charcoal grill or gas grill, place packets on the oiled grill rack directly over medium heat. Cover and grill for 6 to 9 minutes or until fish begins to flake when tested with a fork and zucchini is crisp-tender (carefully open packet to test doneness). Do not turn packets while grilling. Top each serving with sauce.

*Tip: For mango puree, in a blender combine ¼ cup chopped mango and 1 tablespoon water. Cover and blend until smooth. Add any leftover pureed mango to a smoothie.

RIESLING-POACHED COD WITH PESTO-STUFFED TOMATOES

PREP: 30 minutes COOK: 10 minutes MAKES: 4 servings

1 to 1½ pounds fresh or frozen cod fillets, about 1 inch thick
4 roma tomatoes
3 tablespoons Basil Pesto (see recipe)
¼ teaspoon cracked black pepper
1 cup dry Riesling or Sauvignon Blanc
1 sprig fresh thyme or ½ teaspoon dried thyme, crushed
1 bay leaf
½ cup water
2 tablespoons chopped scallion
Lemon wedges

1. Thaw fish, if frozen. Cut tomatoes in half horizontally. Scoop out the seeds and some of the flesh. (If necessary for tomato to sit flat, cut a very thin slice off the end, being careful not to make a hole in the bottom of the tomato.) Spoon some pesto into each tomato half; sprinkle with cracked pepper; set aside.

2. Rinse fish; pat dry with paper towels. Cut fish into four pieces. Place a steamer basket in a large skillet with a tight-fitting lid. Add about ½ inch water to skillet. Bring to boiling; reduce heat to medium. Add the tomatoes, cut sides up, to the basket. Cover and steam for 2 to 3 minutes or until warmed through.

3. Remove tomatoes to a plate; cover to keep warm. Remove steamer basket from skillet; discard water. Add wine, thyme, bay leaf, and the ½ cup water to skillet. Bring to boiling; reduce heat to medium-low. Add fish and scallion.

Simmer, covered, for 8 to 10 minutes or until fish begins to flake when tested with a fork.

4. Drizzle fish with some of the poaching liquid. Serve fish with pesto-stuffed tomatoes and lemon wedges.

BROILED PISTACHIO-CILANTRO-CRUSTED COD OVER SMASHED SWEET POTATOES

PREP: 20 minutes COOK: 10 minutes BROIL: 4 to 6 minutes per ½-inch thickness MAKES: 4 servings

- 1 to 1½ pounds fresh or frozen cod
- Olive oil or refined coconut oil
- 2 tablespoons ground pistachios, pecans, or almonds
- 1 egg white
- ½ teaspoon finely shredded lemon peel
- 1½ pounds sweet potatoes, peeled and cut into chunks
- 2 cloves garlic
- 1 tablespoon coconut oil
- 1 tablespoon grated fresh ginger
- ½ teaspoon ground cumin
- ¼ cup coconut milk (such as Nature's Way)
- 4 teaspoons Cilantro Pesto or Basil Pesto (see recipes)

1. Thaw fish, if frozen. Preheat broiler. Oil rack of a broiler pan. In a small bowl combine ground nuts, egg white, and lemon peel; set aside.

2. For the smashed sweet potatoes, in a medium saucepan cook sweet potatoes and garlic in enough boiling water to cover for 10 to 15 minutes or until tender. Drain; return sweet potatoes and garlic to the saucepan. Using a potato masher, mash sweet potatoes. Stir in 1 tablespoon coconut oil, ginger, and cumin. Mash in coconut milk until light and fluffy.

3. Rinse fish; pat dry with paper towels. Cut fish into four pieces and place on the prepared unheated rack of a

broiler pan. Tuck under any thin edges. Spread each piece with Cilantro Pesto. Spoon nut mixture on pesto and spread gently. Broil fish 4 inches from the heat for 4 to 6 minutes per ½-inch thickness or until fish begins to flake when tested with a fork, covering with foil during broiling if coating starts to burn. Serve fish with sweet potatoes.

ROSEMARY-AND-TANGERINE COD WITH ROASTED BROCCOLI

PREP: 15 minutes MARINATE: up to 30 minutes BAKE: 12 minutes MAKES: 4 servings

1 to 1½ pounds fresh or frozen cod
1 teaspoon finely shredded tangerine peel
½ cup fresh tangerine or orange juice
4 tablespoons olive oil
2 teaspoons snipped fresh rosemary
¼ to ½ teaspoon cracked black pepper
1 teaspoon finely shredded tangerine peel
3 cups broccoli florets
¼ teaspoon crushed red pepper
Tangerine slices, seeds removed

1. Preheat oven to 450°F. Thaw fish, if frozen. Rinse fish; pat dry with paper towels. Cut fish into four serving-size pieces. Measure thickness of fish. In a shallow dish combine tangerine peel, tangerine juice, 2 tablespoons of the olive oil, rosemary, and black pepper; add fish. Cover and marinate in the refrigerator for up to 30 minutes.

2. In a large bowl toss broccoli with the remaining 2 tablespoons olive oil and the crushed red pepper. Place in a 2-quart baking dish.

3. Brush a shallow baking pan lightly with additional olive oil. Drain fish, reserving marinade. Place fish in the pan, tucking under any thin edges. Place fish and broccoli in the oven. Bake broccoli for 12 to 15 minutes or until crisp-tender, stirring once halfway through cooking. Bake fish for 4 to 6 minutes per ½-inch thickness of fish or until fish begins to flake when tested with a fork.

4. In a small saucepan bring reserved marinade to boiling; cook for 2 minutes. Drizzle the marinade over the cooked fish. Serve fish with broccoli and tangerine slices.

CURRIED COD LETTUCE WRAPS WITH PICKLED RADISHES

PREP: 20 minutes STAND: 20 minutes COOK: 6 minutes MAKES: 4 servings PHOTO

1 pound fresh or frozen cod fillets
6 radishes, coarsely shredded
6 to 7 tablespoons cider vinegar
½ teaspoon crushed red pepper
2 tablespoons unrefined coconut oil
¼ cup almond butter
1 clove garlic, minced
2 teaspoons finely grated ginger
2 tablespoons olive oil
1½ to 2 teaspoons no-salt-added curry powder
4 to 8 butterhead lettuce leaves or leaf lettuce leaves
1 red sweet pepper, cut into julienne strips
2 tablespoons snipped fresh cilantro

1. Thaw fish, if frozen. In a medium bowl combine radishes, 4 tablespoons of the vinegar, and ¼ teaspoon of the crushed red pepper; let stand for 20 minutes, stirring occasionally.

2. For almond butter sauce, in a small saucepan melt the coconut oil over low heat. Stir in almond butter until smooth. Stir in garlic, ginger, and remaining ¼ teaspoon crushed red pepper. Remove from heat. Add the remaining 2 to 3 tablespoons cider vinegar, stirring until smooth; set aside. (Sauce will thicken slightly when vinegar is added.)

3. Rinse fish; pat dry with paper towels. In a large skillet heat the olive oil and curry powder over medium heat. Add fish; cook for 3 to 6 minutes or until fish begins to flake

when tested with a fork, turning once halfway through cooking time. Using two forks, coarsely flake fish.

4. Drain radishes; discard marinade. Spoon some of the fish, sweet pepper strips, radish mixture, and almond butter sauce into each lettuce leaf. Sprinkle with cilantro. Wrap leaf around filling. If desired, secure wraps with wooden toothpicks.

ROASTED HADDOCK WITH LEMON AND FENNEL

PREP: 25 minutes ROAST: 50 minutes MAKES: 4 servings

HADDOCK, POLLOCK, AND COD ALL HAVE MILDLY FLAVORED FIRM WHITE FLESH. THEY ARE INTERCHANGEABLE IN MOST RECIPES, INCLUDING THIS SIMPLE DISH OF BAKED FISH AND VEGETABLES WITH HERBS AND WINE.

4 6-ounce fresh or frozen haddock, pollock, or cod fillets, about ½ inch thick
1 large bulb fennel, cored and sliced, fronds reserved and chopped
4 medium carrots, cut in half vertically and sliced into 2- to 3-inch-long pieces
1 red onion, halved and sliced
2 cloves garlic, minced
1 lemon, thinly sliced
3 tablespoons olive oil
½ teaspoon black pepper
¾ cup dry white wine
2 tablespoons finely snipped fresh parsley
2 tablespoons snipped fresh fennel fronds
2 teaspoons finely shredded lemon peel

1. Thaw fish, if frozen. Preheat oven to 400°F. In a 3-quart rectangular baking dish combine fennel, carrots, onion, garlic, and lemon slices. Drizzle with 2 tablespoons of the olive oil and sprinkle with ¼ teaspoon of the pepper; toss to coat. Pour wine into dish. Cover dish with foil.

2. Roast for 20 minutes. Uncover; stir vegetable mixture. Roast 15 to 20 minutes more or until vegetables are crisp-tender. Stir vegetable mixture. Sprinkle fish with the remaining ¼ teaspoon pepper; place fish on top of vegetable mixture. Drizzle with the remaining 1

tablespoon olive oil. Roast about 8 to 10 minutes or until fish begins to flake when tested with a fork.

3. In a small bowl combine parsley, fennel fronds, and lemon peel. To serve, divide fish and vegetable mixture among serving plates. Spoon pan juices over fish and vegetables. Sprinkle with parsley mixture.

PECAN-CRUSTED SNAPPER WITH REMOULADE AND CAJUN-STYLE OKRA AND TOMATOES

PREP: 1 hour COOK: 10 minutes BAKE: 8 minutes MAKES: 4 servings

THIS COMPANY-WORTHY FISH DISH TAKES A BIT OF TIME TO MAKE, BUT THE RICH FLAVORS MAKE IT WELL WORTH IT. THE REMOULADE—A MAYONNAISE-BASED SAUCE SPIKED WITH MUSTARD, LEMON, AND CAJUN SEASONING AND CONFETTIED WITH CHOPPED RED SWEET PEPPER, SCALLIONS, AND PARSLEY—CAN BE MADE A DAY AHEAD AND CHILLED.

- 4 tablespoons olive oil
- ½ cup finely chopped pecans
- 2 tablespoons chopped fresh parsley
- 1 tablespoon chopped fresh thyme
- 2 8-ounce red snapper fillets, ½ inch thick
- 4 teaspoons Cajun Seasoning (see recipe)
- ½ cup diced onion
- ½ cup diced green sweet pepper
- ½ cup diced celery
- 1 tablespoon minced garlic
- 1 pound fresh okra pods, cut into 1-inch-thick slices (or fresh asparagus, cut into 1-inch lengths)
- 8 ounces grape or cherry tomatoes, halved
- 2 teaspoons chopped fresh thyme
- Black pepper
- Rémoulade (see recipe, right)

1. In a medium skillet heat 1 tablespoon of the olive oil over medium heat. Add the pecans and toast about 5 minutes or until golden and fragrant, stirring frequently. Transfer

pecans to a small bowl and let cool. Add parsley and thyme and set aside.

2. Preheat oven to 400°F. Line a baking sheet with parchment paper or foil. Arrange the snapper fillets on the baking sheet, skin sides down, and sprinkle each with 1 teaspoon of the Cajun Seasoning. Using a pastry brush, dab 2 tablespoons of olive oil onto fillets. Divide the pecan mixture evenly among the fillets, pressing the nuts gently onto the surface of the fish so they adhere. Cover all the exposed areas of the fish fillet with nuts if possible. Bake fish for 8 to 10 minutes or until it flakes easily with the tip of a knife.

3. In a large skillet heat the remaining 1 tablespoon olive oil over medium-high heat. Add onion, sweet pepper, celery, and garlic. Cook and stir for 5 minutes or until vegetables are crisp-tender. Add the sliced okra (or asparagus if using) and the tomatoes; cook for 5 to 7 minutes or until okra is crisp-tender and tomatoes begin to split. Remove from heat and season with thyme and black pepper to taste. Serve vegetables with snapper and Rémoulade.

Remoulade: In a food processor pulse ½ cup chopped red sweet pepper, ¼ cup chopped scallions, and 2 tablespoons chopped fresh parsley until fine. Add ¼ cup Paleo Mayo (see recipe), ¼ cup Dijon-Style Mustard (see recipe), 1½ teaspoons lemon juice, and ¼ teaspoon Cajun Seasoning (see recipe). Pulse until combined. Transfer to a serving bowl and refrigerate until ready to serve. (Remoulade may be made 1 day ahead and chilled.)

TARRAGON TUNA PATTIES WITH AVOCADO-LEMON AÏOLI

PREP: 25 minutes COOK: 6 minutes MAKES: 4 servings PHOTO

ALONG WITH SALMON, TUNA IS ONE OF THE RARE KINDS OF FISH THAT CAN BE FINELY CHOPPED AND FORMED INTO BURGERS. BE CAREFUL NOT TO OVERPROCESS THE TUNA IN THE FOOD PROCESSOR—OVERPROCESSING TOUGHENS IT.

1 pound fresh or frozen skinless tuna fillets
1 egg white, lightly beaten
¾ cup ground golden flaxseed meal
1 tablespoon fresh snipped tarragon or dill
2 tablespoons snipped fresh chives
1 teaspoon finely shredded lemon peel
2 tablespoons flaxseed oil, avocado oil, or olive oil
1 medium avocado, seeded
3 tablespoons Paleo Mayo (see recipe)
1 teaspoon finely shredded lemon peel
2 teaspoons fresh lemon juice
1 clove garlic, minced
4 ounces baby spinach (about 4 cups tightly packed)
⅓ cup Roasted Garlic Vinaigrette (see recipe)
1 Granny Smith apple, cored and cut into matchstick-size pieces
¼ cup chopped toasted walnuts (see tip)

1. Thaw fish, if frozen. Rinse fish; pat dry with paper towels. Cut fish into 1½-inch pieces. Place fish in a food processor; process with on/off pulses until finely chopped. (Be careful not to overprocess or you'll toughen the patty.) Set fish aside.

2. In a medium bowl combine egg white, ¼ cup of the flaxseed meal, tarragon, chives, and lemon peel. Add fish; stir gently to combine. Shape fish mixture into four ½-inch-thick patties.

3. Place remaining ½ cup flaxseed meal in a shallow dish. Dip patties into flaxseed mixture, turning to coat evenly.

4. In an extra-large skillet heat oil over medium heat. Cook tuna patties in hot oil for 6 to 8 minutes or until an instant-read thermometer inserted horizontally into patties registers 160°F, turning once halfway through cooking time.

5. Meanwhile, for the aïoli, in a medium bowl use a fork to mash avocado. Add Paleo Mayo, lemon peel, lemon juice, and garlic. Mash until well mixed and almost smooth.

6. Place the spinach in a medium bowl. Drizzle spinach with Roasted Garlic Vinaigrette; toss to coat. For each serving, place a tuna patty and one-fourth of the spinach on a serving plate. Top tuna with some of the aïoli. Top spinach with apple and walnuts. Serve immediately.

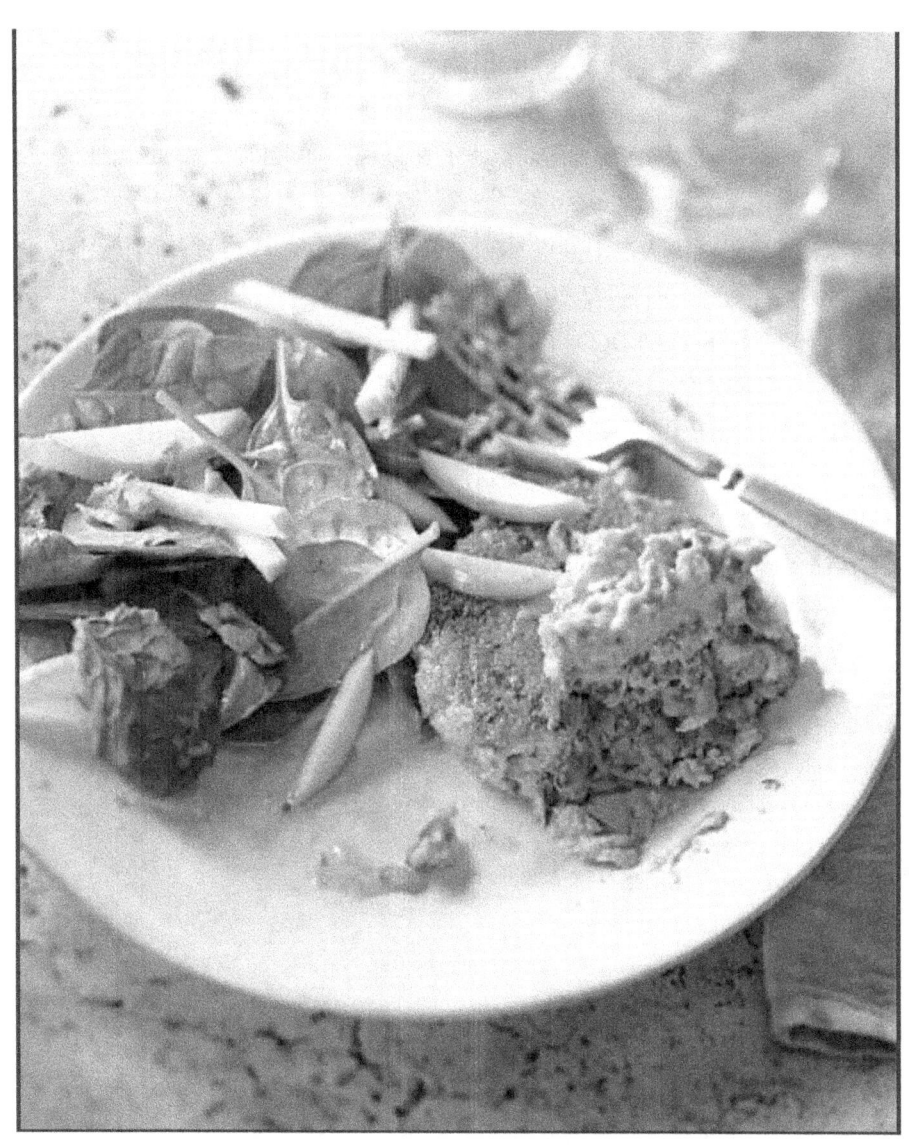

STRIPED BASS TAGINE

PREP: 50 minutes CHILL: 1 to 2 hours COOK: 22 minutes BAKE: 25 minutes MAKES: 4 servings

A TAGINE IS THE NAME OF BOTH A TYPE OF NORTH AFRICAN DISH (A KIND OF STEW) AND THE CONE-SHAPE POT IT'S COOKED IN. IF YOU DON'T HAVE ONE, A COVERED OVEN-GOING SKILLET WORKS JUST FINE. CHERMOULA IS A THICK NORTH AFRICAN HERB PASTE THAT IS MOST OFTEN USED AS A MARINADE FOR FISH. SERVE THIS COLORFUL FISH DISH WITH A SWEET POTATO OR CAULIFLOWER MASH.

- 4 6-ounce fresh or frozen striped bass or halibut fillets, skin on
- 1 bunch cilantro, chopped
- 1 teaspoon finely shredded lemon peel (set aside)
- ¼ cup fresh lemon juice
- 4 tablespoons olive oil
- 5 cloves garlic, minced
- 4 teaspoons ground cumin
- 2 teaspoons sweet paprika
- 1 teaspoon ground coriander
- ¼ teaspoon ground anise
- 1 large onion, peeled, halved, and thinly sliced
- 1 15-ounce can no-salt-added fire-roasted diced tomatoes, undrained
- ½ cup Chicken Bone Broth (see recipe) or no-salt-added chicken broth
- 1 large yellow sweet pepper, seeded and cut into ½-inch- strips
- 1 large orange sweet pepper, seeded and cut into ½-inch strips

1. Thaw fish, if frozen. Rinse fish; pat dry with paper towels. Place fish fillets in a shallow, nonmetal baking dish. Set fish aside.

2. For chermoula, in a blender or small food processor combine cilantro, lemon juice, 2 tablespoons of the olive

oil, 4 cloves minced garlic, the cumin, paprika, coriander, and anise. Cover and process until smooth.

3. Spoon half of the chermoula over the fish, turning fish to coat both sides. Cover and refrigerate for 1 to 2 hours. Cover remaining chermoula; let stand at room temperature until needed.

4. Preheat oven to 325°F. In a large oven-going skillet heat the remaining 2 tablespoons oil over medium-high heat. Add onion; cook and stir for 4 to 5 minutes or until tender. Stir in the remaining 1 clove minced garlic; cook and stir for 1 minute. Add reserved chermoula, tomatoes, Chicken Bone Broth, sweet pepper strips, and lemon peel. Bring to boiling; reduce heat. Simmer, uncovered, for 15 minutes. If desired, transfer mixture to tagine; top with fish and any remaining chermoula from the dish. Cover; bake for 25 minutes. Serve immediately.

HALIBUT IN GARLIC-SHRIMP SAUCE WITH SOFFRITO COLLARD GREENS

PREP: 30 minutes COOK: 19 minutes MAKES: 4 servings

THERE ARE SEVERAL DIFFERENT SOURCES AND TYPES OF HALIBUT, AND THEY CAN BE OF VASTLY DIFFERENT QUALITY—AND FISHED UNDER VERY DIFFERENT CONDITIONS. THE SUSTAINABILITY OF THE FISH, THE ENVIRONMENT IN WHICH IT LIVES, AND THE CONDITIONS UNDER WHICH IT IS RAISED/FISHED ARE ALL FACTORS IN DETERMINING WHICH FISH ARE GOOD CHOICES FOR CONSUMPTION. VISIT THE MONTEREY BAY AQUARIUM WEBSITE (WWW.SEAFOODWATCH.ORG) FOR THE LATEST INFORMATION ON WHICH FISH TO EAT AND WHICH ONES TO AVOID.

4 6-ounce fresh or frozen halibut fillets, about 1 inch thick

Black pepper

6 tablespoons extra virgin olive oil

½ cup finely chopped onion

¼ cup diced red sweet pepper

2 cloves garlic, minced

¾ teaspoon smoked Spanish paprika

½ teaspoon chopped fresh oregano

4 cups collard greens, stemmed, sliced into ¼-inch-thick ribbons (about 12 ounces)

⅓ cup water

8 ounces medium shrimp, peeled, deveined, and coarsely chopped

4 cloves garlic, thinly sliced

¼ to ½ teaspoon crushed red pepper

⅓ cup dry sherry

2 tablespoons lemon juice

¼ cup chopped fresh parsley

1. Thaw fish, if frozen. Rinse fish; pat dry with paper towels. Sprinkle fish with pepper. In a large skillet heat 2 tablespoons of the olive oil over medium heat. Add the fillets; cook for 10 minutes or until golden brown and fish flakes when tested with a fork, turning once halfway through cooking. Transfer the fish to a platter and tent with foil to keep warm.

2. Meanwhile, in another large skillet heat 1 tablespoon of the olive oil over medium heat. Add onion, sweet pepper, 2 cloves minced garlic, paprika, and oregano; cook and stir for 3 to 5 minutes or until tender. Stir in collard greens and the water. Cover and cook for 3 to 4 minutes or until liquid has evaporated and greens are just tender, stirring occasionally. Cover and keep warm until ready to serve.

3. For shrimp sauce, add remaining 3 tablespoons olive oil to the skillet used for cooking the fish. Add the shrimp, 4 cloves sliced garlic, and crushed red pepper. Cook and stir for 2 to 3 minutes or until garlic just begins to turn golden. Add the shrimp; cook for 2 to 3 minutes until shrimp is firm and pink. Stir in the sherry and lemon juice. Cook 1 to 2 minutes or until reduced slightly. Stir in the parsley.

4. Divide shrimp sauce among halibut fillets. Serve with greens.

SEAFOOD BOUILLABAISSE

START TO FINISH: 1¾ hours MAKES: 4 servings

LIKE ITALIAN CIOPPINO, THIS FRENCH SEAFOOD STEW OF FISH AND SHELLFISH SEEMS TO REPRESENT A SAMPLING OF THE DAY'S CATCH THROWN INTO A POT WITH GARLIC, ONIONS, TOMATOES, AND WINE. THE DISTINGUISHING FLAVOR OF BOUILLABAISSE, HOWEVER, IS THE FLAVOR COMBINATION OF SAFFRON, FENNEL, AND ORANGE ZEST.

1 pound fresh or frozen skinless halibut fillet, cut into 1-inch pieces
4 tablespoons olive oil
2 cups chopped onions
4 cloves garlic, smashed
1 head fennel, cored and chopped
6 roma tomatoes, chopped
¾ cup Chicken Bone Broth (see recipe) or no-salt-added chicken broth
¼ cup dry white wine
1 cup finely chopped onion
1 head fennel, cored and finely chopped
6 cloves garlic, minced
1 orange
3 roma tomatoes, finely chopped
4 saffron threads
1 tablespoon snipped fresh oregano
1 pound littleneck clams, scrubbed and rinsed
1 pound mussels, beards removed, scrubbed, and rinsed (see tip)
Snipped fresh oregano (optional)

1. Thaw halibut, if frozen. Rinse fish; pat dry with paper towels. Set fish aside.

2. In a 6- to 8-quart Dutch oven, heat 2 tablespoons of the olive oil over medium heat. Add 2 cups chopped onions , 1 head

chopped fennel, and 4 cloves smashed garlic to the pot. Cook for 7 to 9 minutes or until onion is tender, stirring occasionally. Add 6 chopped tomatoes and 1 head chopped fennel; cook for 4 minutes more. Add Chicken Bone Broth and white wine to pot; simmer for 5 minutes; cool slightly. Transfer vegetable mixture to a blender or food processor. Cover and blend or process until smooth; set aside.

3. In the same Dutch oven heat the remaining 1 tablespoon olive oil over medium heat. Add 1 cup finely chopped onion, 1 head finely chopped fennel, and 6 cloves minced garlic. Cook over medium heat 5 to 7 minutes or until nearly tender, stirring frequently.

4. Use a vegetable peeler to remove the zest from the orange in wide strips; set aside. Add the pureed vegetable mixture, 3 chopped tomatoes, saffron, oregano, and orange zest strips to the Dutch oven. Bring to boiling; reduce heat to maintain simmering. Add clams, mussels, and fish; stir gently to coat fish with sauce. Adjust heat as needned to maintain a simmer. Cover and simmer gently for 3 to 5 minutes until mussels and clams have opened and fish begins to flake when tested with a fork. Ladle into shallow bowls to serve. If desired, sprinkle with additional oregano.

CLASSIC SHRIMP CEVICHE

PREP: 20 minutes COOK: 2 minutes CHILL: 1 hour STAND: 30 minutes MAKES: 3 to 4 servings

THIS LATIN AMERICAN DISH IS AN EXPLOSION OF TASTES AND TEXTURES. CRUNCHY CUCUMBER AND CELERY, CREAMY AVOCADO, HOT AND SPICY JALAPEÑOS, AND DELICATE, SWEET SHRIMP INTERMINGLE IN LIME JUICE AND OLIVE OIL. IN TRADITIONAL CEVICHE, THE ACID IN THE LIME JUICE "COOKS" THE SHRIMP—BUT A QUICK DIP IN BOILING WATER LEAVES NOTHING TO CHANCE, SAFETYWISE—AND DOESN'T HURT THE FLAVOR OR TEXTURE OF THE SHRIMP.

- 1 pound fresh or frozen medium shrimp, peeled and deveined, tails removed
- ½ of a cucumber, peeled, seeded, and chopped
- 1 cup chopped celery
- ½ of a small red onion, chopped
- 1 to 2 jalapeños, seeded and minced (see tip)
- ½ cup fresh lime juice
- 2 roma tomatoes, diced
- 1 avocado, halved, seeded, peeled, and diced
- ¼ cup snipped fresh cilantro
- 3 tablespoons olive oil
- ½ teaspoon black pepper

1. Thaw shrimp, if frozen. Peel and devein shrimp; remove tails. Rinse shrimp; pat dry with paper towels.

2. Fill a large saucepan half full with water. Bring to boiling. Add shrimp to boiling water. Cook, uncovered, for 1 to 2 minutes or just until shrimp turn opaque; drain. Run shrimp under cool water and drain again. Dice shrimp.

3. In a extra-large nonreactive bowl combine shrimp, cucumber, celery, onion, jalapeños, and lime juice. Cover and refrigerate for 1 hour, stirring once or twice.

4. Stir in tomatoes, avocado, cilantro, olive oil, and black pepper. Cover and let stand at room temperature for 30 minutes. Stir gently before serving.

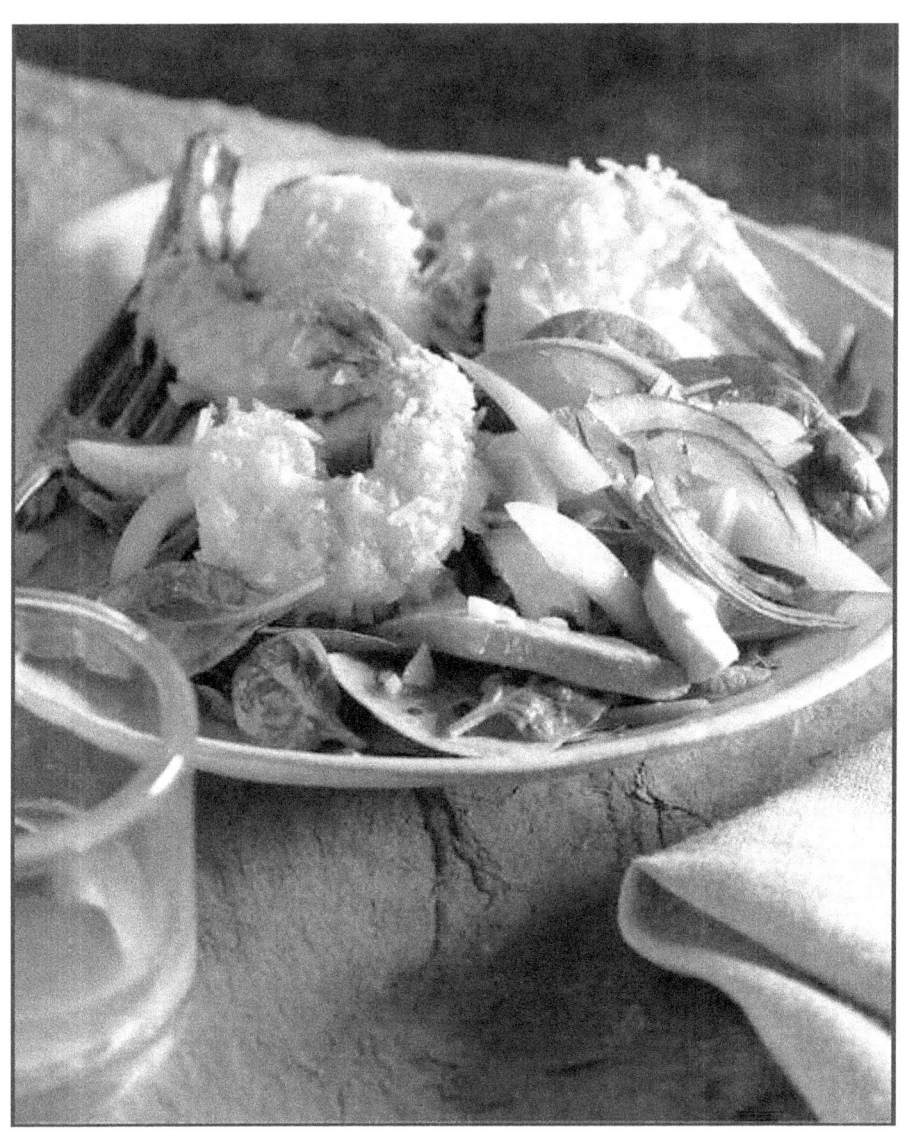

COCONUT-CRUSTED SHRIMP AND SPINACH SALAD

PREP: 25 minutes BAKE: 8 minutes MAKES: 4 servings PHOTO

COMMERCIALLY PRODUCED CANS OF SPRAY OLIVE OIL CAN CONTAIN GRAIN ALCOHOL, LECITHIN, AND PROPELLANT—NOT A TERRIFIC MIX WHEN YOU ARE TRYING TO EAT PURE, REAL FOODS AND AVOID GRAINS, UNHEALTHY FATS, LEGUMES, AND DAIRY. AN OIL MISTER USES ONLY AIR TO PROPEL THE OIL INTO A FINE SPRAY—PERFECT FOR LIGHTLY COATING COCONUT-CRUSTED SHRIMP BEFORE BAKING.

1½ pounds fresh or frozen extra-large shrimp in shells
Misto spray bottle filled with extra virgin olive oil
2 eggs
¾ cup unsweetened flaked or shredded coconut
¾ cup almond meal
½ cup avocado oil or olive oil
3 tablespoons fresh lemon juice
2 tablespoons fresh lime juice
2 small cloves garlic, minced
⅛ to ¼ teaspoon crushed red pepper
8 cups fresh baby spinach
1 medium avocado, halved, seeded, peeled, and thinly sliced
1 small orange or yellow sweet pepper, cut into thin bite-size strips
½ cup slivered red onion

1. Thaw shrimp, if frozen. Peel and devein shrimp, leaving tails intact. Rinse shrimp; pat dry with paper towels. Preheat oven to 450°F. Line a large baking sheet with foil; lightly coat foil with oil sprayed from the Misto bottle; set aside.

2. In a shallow dish beat eggs with a fork. In another shallow dish combine coconut and almond meal. Dip shrimp into eggs, turning to coat. Dip in coconut mixture, pressing to coat (leave tails uncoated). Arrange shrimp in a single layer on the prepared baking sheet. Coat the tops of the shrimp with oil sprayed from the Misto bottle.

3. Bake for 8 to 10 minutes or until shrimp are opaque and coating is lightly browned.

4. Meanwhile, for dressing, in a small screw-top jar combine avocado oil, lemon juice, lime juice, garlic, and crushed red pepper. Cover and shake well.

5. For salads, divide spinach among four serving plates. Top with avocado, sweet pepper, red onion, and the shrimp. Drizzle with dressing and serve immediately.

TROPICAL SHRIMP AND SCALLOP CEVICHE

PREP: 20 minutes MARINATE: 30 to 60 minutes MAKES: 4 to 6 servings

COOL AND LIGHT CEVICHE MAKES A GREAT MEAL FOR A HOT SUMMER NIGHT. WITH MELON, MANGO, SERRANO CHILES, FENNEL, AND MANGO-LIME SALAD DRESSING (SEE RECIPE), THIS IS A SWEET-HOT TAKE ON THE ORIGINAL.

1 pound fresh or frozen sea scallops
1 pound fresh or frozen large shrimp
2 cups cubed honeydew melon
2 medium mangoes, pitted, peeled, and chopped (about 2 cups)
1 head fennel, trimmed, quartered, cored, and thinly sliced
1 medium red sweet pepper, chopped (about ¾ cup)
1 to 2 serrano chiles, seeded if desired and thinly sliced (see tip)
½ cup lightly packed fresh cilantro, chopped
1 recipe Mango-Lime Salad Dressing (see recipe)

1. Thaw scallops and shrimp, if frozen. Split scallops in half horizontally. Peel, devein, and split shrimp in half horizontally. Rinse scallops and shrimp; pat dry with paper towels. Fill a large saucepan three-fourths full with water. Bring to boiling. Add shrimp and scallops; cook for 3 to 4 minutes or until shrimp and scallops are opaque; drain and rinse with cold water to cool quickly. Drain well and set aside.

2. In an extra-large bowl combine melon, mangoes, fennel, sweet pepper, serrano chiles, and cilantro. Add Mango-Lime Salad Dressing; toss gently to coat. Gently stir in

cooked shrimp and scallops. Marinate in the refrigerator for 30 to 60 minutes before serving.

JAMAICAN JERK SHRIMP WITH AVOCADO OIL

START TO FINISH: 20 minutes MAKES: 4 servings

WITH A TOTAL TO-THE-TABLE TIME OF 20 MINUTES, THIS DISH OFFERS ONE MORE COMPELLING REASON TO EAT A HEALTHY MEAL AT HOME, EVEN ON THE BUSIEST NIGHTS.

1 pound fresh or frozen medium shrimp
1 cup chopped, peeled mango (1 medium)
⅓ cup thinly sliced red onion sliced
¼ cup snipped fresh cilantro
1 tablespoon fresh lime juice
2 to 3 tablespoons Jamaican Jerk Seasoning (see recipe)
1 tablespoons extra virgin olive oil
2 tablespoons avocado oil

1. Thaw shrimp, if frozen. In a medium bowl stir together mango, onion, cilantro, and lime juice.

2. Peel and devein shrimp. Rinse shrimp; pat dry with paper towels. Place shrimp in a medium bowl. Sprinkle with Jamaican Jerk Seasoning; toss to coat shrimp on all sides.

3. In a large nonstick skillet heat olive oil over medium-high heat. Add shrimp; cook and stir about 4 minutes or until opaque. Drizzle shrimp with avocado oil and serve with the mango mixture.

SHRIMP SCAMPI WITH WILTED SPINACH AND RADICCHIO

PREP: 15 minutes COOK: 8 minutes MAKES: 3 servings

"SCAMPI" REFERS TO A CLASSIC RESTAURANT DISH OF LARGE SHRIMP SAUTÉED OR BROILED WITH BUTTER AND LOTS OF GARLIC AND LEMON. THIS SPICY OLIVE OIL VERSION IS PALEO-APPROVED—AND BUMPED UP NUTRITIONALLY WITH A QUICK SAUTÉ OF RADICCHIO AND SPINACH.

1 pound fresh or frozen large shrimp
4 tablespoons extra virgin olive oil
6 cloves garlic, minced
½ teaspoon black pepper
¼ cup dry white wine
½ cup snipped fresh parsley
½ of a head radicchio, cored and thinly sliced
½ teaspoon crushed red pepper
9 cups baby spinach
Lemon wedges

1. Thaw shrimp, if frozen. Peel and devein shrimp, leaving tails intact. In a large skillet heat 2 tablespoons of the olive oil over medium-high heat. Add shrimp, 4 cloves minced garlic, and black pepper. Cook and stir about 3 minutes or until shrimp are opaque. Transfer shrimp mixture to a bowl.

2. Add white wine to skillet. Cook, stirring to loosen to any browned garlic from bottom of the skillet. Pour wine over shrimp; toss to combine. Stir in parsley. Cover loosely with foil to keep warm; set aside.

3. Add the remaining 2 tablespoons olive oil, the remaining 2 cloves minced garlic, the radicchio, and crushed red pepper to the skillet. Cook and stir over medium heat for 3 minutes or until radicchio just begins to wilt. Carefully stir in the spinach; cook and stir for 1 to 2 minutes more or until spinach is just wilted.

4. To serve, divide spinach mixture among three serving plates; top with shrimp mixture. Serve with lemon wedges for squeezing over shrimp and greens.

CRAB SALAD WITH AVOCADO, GRAPEFRUIT, AND JICAMA

START TO FINISH: 30 minutes MAKES: 4 servings

JUMBO LUMP OR BACKFIN CRABMEAT IS BEST FOR THIS SALAD. JUMBO LUMP CRABMEAT IS MADE UP OF LARGE CHUNKS THAT WORK WELL IN SALADS. BACKFIN IS A BLEND OF BROKEN PIECES OF JUMBO LUMP CRABMEAT AND SMALLER PIECES OF CRABMEAT FROM THE BODY OF THE CRAB. ALTHOUGH SMALLER THAN THE JUMBO LUMP CRAB, BACKFIN WORKS JUST FINE. FRESH IS BEST, OF COURSE, BUT THAWED FROZEN CRAB IS A FINE OPTION.

6 cups baby spinach

½ of a medium jicama, peeled and julienne-cut*

2 pink or ruby red grapefruit, peeled, seeded, and sectioned**

2 small avocados, halved

1 pound jumbo lump or backfin crabmeat

Basil-Grapefruit Dressing (see recipe, right)

1. Divide spinach among four serving plates. Top with jicama, grapefruit sections and any accumulated juice, avocados, and crabmeat. Drizzle with Basil-Grapefruit Dressing.

Basil-Grapefruit Dressing: In a screw-top jar combine ⅓ cup extra virgin olive oil; ¼ cup fresh grapefruit juice; 2 tablespoons fresh orange juice; ½ of a small shallot, minced; 2 tablespoons finely snipped fresh basil; ¼ teaspoon crushed red pepper; and ¼ teaspoon black pepper. Cover and shake well.

*Tip: A julienne peeler makes quick work of cutting the jicama into thin strips.

**Tip: To section grapefruit, cut a slice off the stem end and bottom of the fruit. Set it upright on a work surface. Cut down the fruit in sections from top to bottom, following the rounded shape of the fruit, to remove peel in strips. Hold the fruit over a bowl and, using a paring knife, cut to the center of the fruit on the sides of each segment to release it from the pith. Place segments in bowl with any accumulated juices. Discard pith.

CAJUN LOBSTER TAIL BOIL WITH TARRAGON AÏOLI

PREP: 20 minutes COOK: 30 minutes MAKES: 4 servings PHOTO

FOR A ROMANTIC DINNER FOR TWO, THIS RECIPE IS EASILY CUT IN HALF. USE VERY SHARP KITCHEN SHEARS TO CUT OPEN THE SHELL OF THE LOBSTER TAILS AND GET AT THE RICHLY FLAVORED MEAT.

2 recipes Cajun Seasoning (see recipe)
12 cloves garlic, peeled and halved
2 lemons, halved
2 large carrots, peeled
2 celery stalks, peeled
2 fennel bulbs, sliced into thin wedges
1 pound whole button mushrooms
4 7- to 8-ounce Maine lobster tails
4 8-inch bamboo skewers
½ cup Paleo Aïoli (Garlic Mayo) (see recipe)
¼ cup Dijon-Style Mustard (see recipe)
2 tablespoons snipped fresh tarragon or parsley

1. In an 8-quart stockpot combine 6 cups water, Cajun Seasoning, garlic, and lemons. Bring to boiling; boil for 5 minutes. Reduce heat to keep liquid at a simmer.

2. Cut the carrots and celery crosswise into four pieces. Add carrots, celery, and fennel to liquid. Cover and cook for 10 minutes. Add mushrooms; cover and cook for 5 minutes. Using a slotted spoon, transfer vegetables to a serving bowl; keep warm.

3. Starting from the body end of each lobster tail, slide a skewer between the meat and the shell, going almost all the way through the tail end. (This will keep the tail from curling as it cooks.) Reduce heat. Cook lobster tails in the barely simmering liquid in pot for 8 to 12 minutes or until shells turn bright red and meat is tender when pierced with a fork. Remove lobster from cooking liquid. Use a kitchen towel to hold the lobster tails and remove and discard the skewers.

4. In a small bowl stir together the Paleo Aïoli, Dijon-Style Mustard, and tarragon. Serve with the lobster and vegetables.

MUSSELS FRITES WITH SAFFRON AÏOLI

START TO FINISH: 1¼ hours MAKES: 4 servings

THIS IS A PALEO TAKE ON THE FRENCH CLASSIC OF MUSSELS STEAMED IN WHITE WINE AND HERBS AND SERVED WITH THIN AND CRISPY FRITES MADE FROM WHITE POTATOES. DISCARD ANY MUSSELS THAT WON'T CLOSE BEFORE THEY'RE COOKED—AND ANY MUSSELS THAT DON'T OPEN AFTER THEY'RE COOKED.

PARSNIP FRITES

- 1½ pounds parsnips, peeled and cut into 3×¼-inch julienne
- 3 tablespoons olive oil
- 2 cloves garlic, minced
- ¼ teaspoon black pepper
- ⅛ teaspoon cayenne pepper

SAFFRON AÏOLI

- ⅓ cup Paleo Aïoli (Garlic Mayo) (see recipe)
- ⅛ teaspoon saffron threads, gently crushed

MUSSELS

- 4 tablespoons olive oil
- ½ cup finely chopped shallots
- 6 cloves garlic, minced
- ¼ teaspoon black pepper
- 3 cups dry white wine
- 3 large sprigs flat-leaf parsley
- 4 pounds mussels, cleaned and debearded*
- ¼ cup chopped fresh Italian (flat-leaf) parsley
- 2 tablespoons snipped fresh tarragon (optional)

1. For parsnip frites, preheat oven to 450°F. Soak cut parsnips in enough cold water to cover in the refrigerator for 30 minutes; drain and pat dry with paper towels.

2. Line a large baking sheet with parchment paper. Place parsnips in an extra-large bowl. In a small bowl combine 3 tablespoons olive oil, 2 cloves minced garlic, ¼ teaspoon black pepper, and cayenne pepper; drizzle over parsnips and toss to coat. Arrange parsnips in an even layer on prepared baking sheet. Bake for 30 to 35 minutes or tender and starting to brown, stirring occasionally.

3. For aïoli, in a small bowl stir together Paleo Aïoli and saffron. Cover and refrigerate until serving time.

4. Meanwhile, in a 6- to 8-quart stockpot or Dutch oven heat the 4 tablespoons olive oil over medium heat. Add shallots, 6 cloves garlic, and ¼ teaspoon black pepper; cook about 2 minutes or until soft and wilted, stirring frequently.

5. Add wine and parsley sprigs to pot; bring to boiling. Add mussels, stirring a few times. Cover tightly and steam for 3 to 5 minutes or until shells open, gently stirring twice. Discard any mussels that do not open.

6. With a large skimmer, transfer mussels into shallow soup dishes. Remove and discard parsley sprigs from cooking liquid; ladle cooking liquid over the mussels. Sprinkle with chopped parsley and, if desired, tarragon. Serve immediately with parsnip frites and saffron aïoli.

*Tip: Cook mussels the day they are purchased. If using wild-harvested mussels, soak in a bowl of cold water for 20 minutes to help flush out grit and sand. (This is not necessary for farm-raised mussels.) Using a stiff brush, scrub mussels, one at a time, under cold running water. Debeard mussels about 10 to 15 minutes before cooking. The beard is the small cluster of fibers that emerge from the shell. To remove the beards, grasp the string between your thumb and forefinger and yank toward the hinge. (This method will not kill the mussel.) You can also use pliers or fish tweezers. Be sure that the shell of each mussel is tightly closed. If any shells are open, tap them gently on the counter. Discard any mussels that don't close within a few minutes. Discard any mussels with cracked or damaged shells.

SEARED SCALLOPS WITH BEET RELISH

START TO FINISH: 30 minutes MAKES: 4 servings PHOTO

FOR A BEAUTIFUL GOLDEN CRUST, BE SURE THE SURFACE OF THE SCALLOPS IS REALLY DRY—AND THAT THE PAN IS NICE AND HOT—BEFORE ADDING THEM TO THE PAN. ALSO, LET THE SCALLOPS SEAR WITHOUT DISTURBING THEM FOR 2 TO 3 MINUTES, CAREFULLY CHECKING BEFORE TURNING.

1 pound fresh or frozen sea scallops, patted dry with paper towels
3 medium red beets, peeled and cut chopped
½ of a Granny Smith apple, peeled and chopped
2 jalapeños, stemmed, seeded, and minced (see tip)
¼ cup chopped fresh cilantro
2 tablespoons finely chopped red onion
4 tablespoons olive oil
2 tablespoons fresh lime juice
White pepper

1. Thaw scallops, if frozen.

2. For beet relish, in a medium bowl combine beets, apple, jalapeños, cilantro, onion, 2 tablespoons of the olive oil, and lime juice. Mix well. Set aside while preparing scallops.

3. Rinse scallops; pat dry with paper towels. In a large skillet heat the remaining 2 tablespoons olive oil over medium-high heat. Add scallops; sauté for 4 to 6 minutes or until golden brown on the exterior and barely opaque. Sprinkle scallops lightly with white pepper.

4. To serve, divide beet relish evenly among serving plates; top with scallops. Serve immediately.

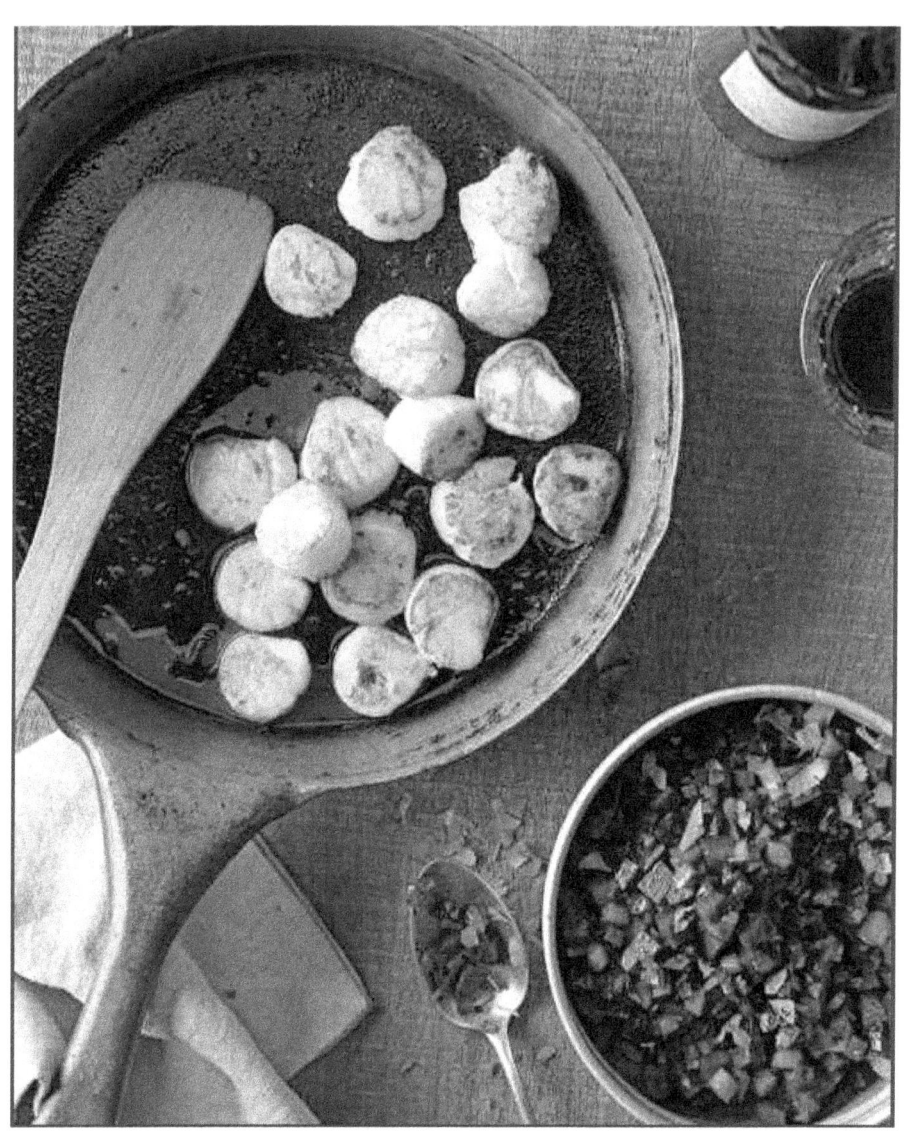

GRILLED SCALLOPS WITH CUCUMBER-DILL SALSA

PREP: 35 minutes CHILL: 1 to 24 hours GRILL: 9 minutes MAKES: 4 servings

HERE'S A TIP FOR GETTING THE MOST FLAWLESS AVOCADOS: BUY THEM WHEN THEY ARE BRIGHT GREEN AND HARD, THEN RIPEN THEM ON THE COUNTER FOR A FEW DAYS—UNTIL THEY GIVE JUST SLIGHTLY WHEN LIGHTLY PRESSED WITH YOUR FINGERS. WHEN HARD AND UNRIPE, THEY WON'T BRUISE IN TRANSIT FROM THE MARKET.

12 or 16 fresh or frozen sea scallops (1¼ to 1¾ pounds total)
¼ cup olive oil
4 cloves garlic, minced
1 teaspoon freshly ground black pepper
2 medium zucchini, trimmed and halved lengthwise
½ of a medium cucumber, halved lengthwise and thinly sliced crosswise
1 medium avocado, halved, seeded, peeled, and chopped
1 medium tomato, cored, seeded, and chopped
2 teaspoons snipped fresh mint
1 teaspoon snipped fresh dill

1. Thaw scallops, if frozen. Rinse scallops with cold water; pat dry with paper towels. In a large bowl combine 3 tablespoons of the oil, the garlic, and ¾ teaspoon of the pepper. Add scallops; toss gently to coat. Cover and chill for at least 1 hour or up to 24 hours, gently stirring occasionally.

2. Brush zucchini halves with the remaining 1 tablespoon oil; sprinkle evenly with remaining ¼ teaspoon pepper.

3. Drain scallops, discarding marinade. Thread two 10- to 12-inch skewers through each scallop, using 3 or 4 scallops for each pair of skewers and leaving a ½-inch space between scallops.* (Threading the scallops on two skewers helps keep them stable when grilling and turning.)

4. For a charcoal or gas grill, place scallop kabobs and zucchini halves on the grill rack directly over medium heat.** Cover and grill until scallops are opaque and zucchini are just tender, turning halfway through grilling. Allow 6 to 8 minutes for scallops and 9 to 11 minutes for zucchini.

5. Meanwhile, for salsa, in a medium bowl combine cucumber, avocado, tomato, mint, and dill. Toss gently to combine. Place 1 scallop kabob on each of four serving plates. Diagonally cut zucchini halves crosswise in half and add to plates with scallops. Spoon cucumber mixture evenly over scallops.

*Tip: If using wooden skewers, soak in enough water to cover for 30 minutes before using.

**To broil: Prepare as directed through Step 3. Place scallop kabobs and zucchini halves on the unheated rack of a broiler pan. Broil 4 to 5 inches from the heat until scallops are opaque and zucchini is just tender, turning once halfway through cooking. Allow 6 to 8 minutes for scallops and 10 to 12 minutes for zucchini.

SEARED SCALLOPS WITH TOMATO, OLIVE OIL, AND HERB SAUCE

PREP: 20 minutes COOK: 4 minutes MAKES: 4 servings

THE SAUCE IS ALMOST LIKE A WARM VINAIGRETTE. OLIVE OIL, CHOPPED FRESH TOMATO, LEMON JUICE, AND HERBS ARE COMBINED AND VERY GENTLY HEATED—JUST ENOUGH TO MELD THE FLAVORS—AND THEN SERVED WITH THE SEARED SCALLOPS AND A CRUNCHY SUNFLOWER SPROUT SALAD.

SCALLOPS AND SAUCE
- 1 to 1½ pounds large fresh or frozen sea scallops (about 12)
- 2 large roma tomatoes, peeled,* seeded, and chopped
- ½ cup olive oil
- 2 tablespoons fresh lemon juice
- 2 tablespoons snipped fresh basil
- 1 to 2 teaspoons finely chopped chives
- 1 tablespoon olive oil

SALAD
- 4 cups sunflower sprouts
- 1 lemon, cut into wedges
- Extra virgin olive oil

1. Thaw scallops, if frozen. Rinse scallops; pat dry. Set aside.

2. For sauce, in a small saucepan combine tomatoes, ½ cup olive oil, the lemon juice, basil, and chives; set aside.

3. In a large skillet heat the 1 tablespoon olive oil over medium-high heat. Add scallops; cook for 4 to 5 minutes or until browned and opaque, turning once halfway through cooking.

4. For the salad, place the sprouts in a serving bowl. Squeeze lemon wedges over sprouts and drizzle with a little olive oil. Toss to combine.

5. Heat the sauce over low heat until warm; do not boil. To serve, spoon some of the sauce in the center of the plate; top with 3 of the scallops. Serve with the sprouts salad.

*Tip: To easily peel a tomato, drop the tomato into a pot of boiling water for 30 seconds to 1 minute or until the skin starts to split. Remove tomato from the boiling water and immediately plunge into a bowl of ice water to stop the cooking process. When tomato is cool enough to handle, slip the skin off.

CUMIN-ROASTED CAULIFLOWER WITH FENNEL AND PEARL ONIONS

PREP: 15 minutes COOK: 25 minutes MAKES: 4 servings PHOTO

THERE IS SOMETHING PARTICULARLY ENTICING ABOUT THE COMBINATION OF ROASTED CAULIFLOWER AND THE TOASTY, EARTHY TASTE OF CUMIN. THIS DISH HAS THE ADDITIONAL ELEMENT OF SWEETNESS FROM DRIED CURRANTS. IF YOU LIKE, YOU COULD ADD A LITTLE HEAT WITH ¼ TO ½ TEASPOON OF CRUSHED RED PEPPER ALONG WITH THE CUMIN AND CURRANTS IN STEP 2.

3 tablespoons unrefined coconut oil
1 medium head cauliflower, cut into florets (4 to 5 cups)
2 heads fennel, coarsely chopped
1½ cups frozen pearl onions, thawed and drained
¼ cup dried currants
2 teaspoons ground cumin
Snipped fresh dill (optional)

1. In an extra-large skillet heat coconut oil over medium heat. Add cauliflower, fennel, and pearl onions. Cover and cook for 15 minutes, stirring occasionally.

2. Reduce heat to medium-low. Add currants and cumin to skillet; cook, uncovered, about 10 minutes or until cauliflower and fennel are tender and golden brown. If desired, garnish with dill.

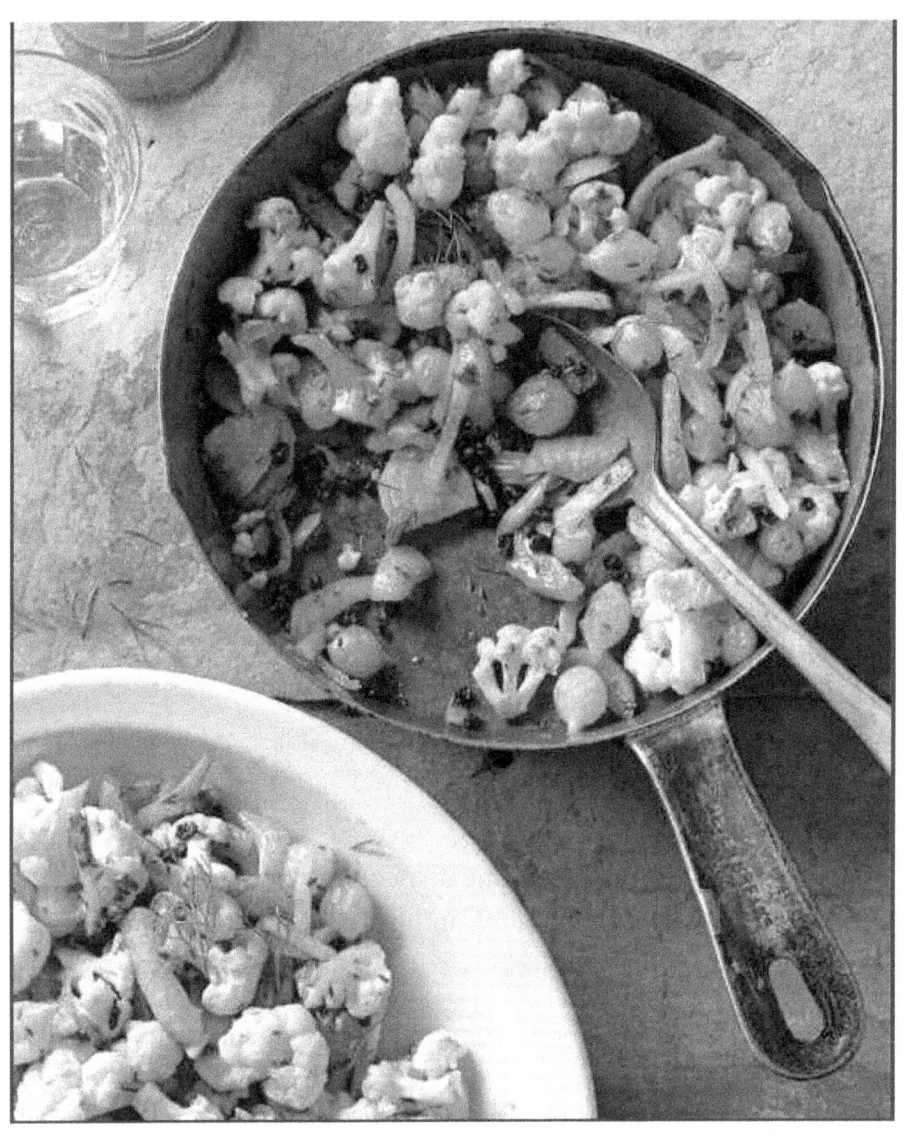

CHUNKY TOMATO-EGGPLANT SAUCE WITH SPAGHETTI SQUASH

PREP: 30 minutes BAKE: 50 minutes COOL: 10 minutes COOK: 10 minutes MAKES: 4 servings

THIS SAUCY SIDE DISH IS EASILY TURNED INTO A MAIN DISH. ADD ABOUT 1 POUND OF COOKED GROUND BEEF OR BISON TO THE EGGPLANT-TOMATO MIXTURE AFTER YOU MASH IT LIGHTLY WITH A POTATO MASHER.

1 2- to 2½-pound spaghetti squash
2 tablespoons olive oil
1 cup chopped, peeled eggplant
¾ cup chopped onion
1 small red sweet pepper, chopped (½ cup)
4 cloves garlic, minced
4 medium red ripe tomatoes, peeled if desired and coarsely chopped (about 2 cups)
½ cup torn fresh basil

1. Preheat oven to 375°F. Line a small baking pan with parchment paper. Cut spaghetti squash in half crosswise. Use a large spoon to scrape out any seeds and strings. Place squash halves, cut sides down, on prepared baking sheet. Bake, uncovered, for 50 to 60 minutes or until squash is tender. Cool on a wire rack about 10 minutes.

2. Meanwhile, in a large skillet heat olive oil over medium heat. Add onion, eggplant and pepper; cook for 5 to 7 minutes or until vegetables are tender, stirring occasionally. Add garlic; cook and stir 30 seconds more. Add tomatoes; cook for 3 to 5 minutes or until tomatoes are softened, stirring occasionally. Using a potato masher,

mash the mixture lightly. Stir in half the basil. Cover and cook for 2 minutes.

3. Use a pot holder or towel to hold squash halves. Use a fork to scrape the squash pulp into a medium bowl. Divide squash among four serving plates. Top evenly with sauce. Sprinkle with remaining basil.

STUFFED PORTOBELLO MUSHROOMS

PREP: 35 minutes BAKE: 20 minutes COOK: 7 minutes MAKES: 4 servings

TO GET THE FRESHEST PORTOBELLOS, LOOK FOR MUSHROOMS THAT STILL HAVE THEIR STEMS INTACT. THE GILLS SHOULD LOOK MOIST BUT NOT WET OR BLACK AND SHOULD HAVE GOOD SEPARATION BETWEEN THEM. TO PREPARE ANY KIND OF MUSHROOMS FOR COOKING, WIPE WITH A SLIGHTLY DAMP PAPER TOWEL. NEVER RUN MUSHROOMS UNDER WATER OR SOAK THEM IN WATER—THEY ARE HIGHLY ABSORBENT AND WILL GET MUSHY AND WATERLOGGED.

4 large portobello mushrooms (about 1 pound total)
¼ cup olive oil
1 tablespoon Smoky Seasoning (see recipe)
2 tablespoons olive oil
½ cup chopped shallots
1 tablespoon minced garlic
1 pound Swiss chard, stemmed and chopped (about 10 cups)
2 teaspoons Mediterranean Seasoning (see recipe)
½ cup chopped radishes

1. Preheat oven to 400°F. Remove stems from mushrooms and reserve for Step 2. Use the tip of a spoon to scrape the gills out of the caps; discard gills. Place mushroom caps in a 3-quart rectangular baking dish; brush both sides of mushrooms with the ¼ cup olive oil. Turn mushroom caps so the stemmed sides are up; sprinkle with Smoky Seasoning. Cover baking dish with foil. Bake, covered, about 20 minutes or until tender.

2. Meanwhile, chop reserved mushroom stems; set aside. To prepare chard, remove thick ribs from leaves and discard. Coarsely chop the chard leaves.

3. In an extra-large skillet heat the 2 tablespoons olive oil over medium heat. Add shallots and garlic; cook and stir for 30 seconds. Add chopped mushroom stems, chopped chard, and Mediterranean Seasoning. Cook, uncovered, for 6 to 8 minutes or until chard is tender, stirring occasionally.

4. Divide chard mixture among the mushroom caps. Drizzle any liquid remaining in baking dish over stuffed mushrooms. Top with chopped radishes.

ROASTED RADICCHIO

PREP: 20 minutes COOK: 15 minutes MAKES: 4 servings

RADICCHIO IS MOST OFTEN EATEN AS PART OF A SALAD TO PROVIDE A PLEASANT BITTERNESS AMONG THE MIX OF GREENS—BUT IT CAN BE ROASTED OR GRILLED ON ITS OWN AS WELL. A SLIGHT BITTERNESS IS INHERENT TO RADICCHIO, BUT YOU DON'T WANT IT TO BE OVERWHELMING. LOOK FOR SMALLER HEADS WHOSE LEAVES LOOK FRESH AND CRISP—NOT WILTED. THE CUT END MAY BE A LITTLE BROWN BUT SHOULD BE MOSTLY WHITE. IN THIS RECIPE, A SPLASH OF BALSAMIC VINEGAR BEFORE SERVING ADDS A HINT OF SWEETNESS.

2 large heads radicchio

¼ cup olive oil

1 teaspoon Mediterranean Seasoning (see recipe)

¼ cup balsamic vinegar

1. Preheat oven to 400°F. Quarter the radicchio, leaving some of the core attached (you should have 8 wedges). Brush cut sides of radicchio wedges with olive oil. Place wedges, cut sides down, on a baking sheet; sprinkle with Mediterranean Seasoning.

2. Roast about 15 minutes or until radicchio wilts, turning once halfway through roasting. Arrange radicchio on a serving platter. Drizzle balsamic vinegar; serve immediately.

ROASTED FENNEL WITH ORANGE VINAIGRETTE

PREP: 25 minutes ROAST: 25 minutes MAKES: 4 servings

SAVE ANY LEFTOVER VINAIGRETTE TO TOSS WITH SALAD GREENS—OR SERVE WITH GRILLED PORK, POULTRY, OR FISH. STORE LEFTOVER VINAIGRETTE IN A TIGHTLY COVERED CONTAINER IN THE REFRIGERATOR FOR UP TO 3 DAYS.

6 tablespoons extra virgin olive oil, plus more for brushing

1 large fennel bulb, trimmed, cored, and cut into wedges (reserve fronds for garnish if desired)

1 red onion, cut into wedges

½ of an orange, thinly sliced into rounds

½ cup orange juice

2 tablespoons white wine vinegar or champagne vinegar

2 tablespoons apple cider

1 teaspoon ground fennel seeds

1 teaspoon finely shredded orange peel

½ teaspoon Dijon-Style Mustard (see recipe)

Black pepper

1. Preheat oven to 425°F. Brush a large baking sheet lightly with olive oil. Arrange the fennel, onion, and orange slices on the baking sheet; drizzle with 2 tablespoons of the olive oil. Gently toss vegetable to coat with oil.

2. Roast vegetables for 25 to 30 minutes or until vegetables are tender and light golden, turning once halfway through roasting.

3. Meanwhile, for orange vinaigrette, in a blender combine orange juice, vinegar, apple cider, fennel seeds, orange

peel, Dijon-Style Mustard, and pepper to taste. With the blender running, slowly add the remaining 4 tablespoons olive oil in a thin stream. Continue blending until vinaigrette thickens.

4. Transfer vegetables to a serving platter. Drizzle vegetables with some of the vinaigrette. If desired, garnish with reserved fennel fronds.

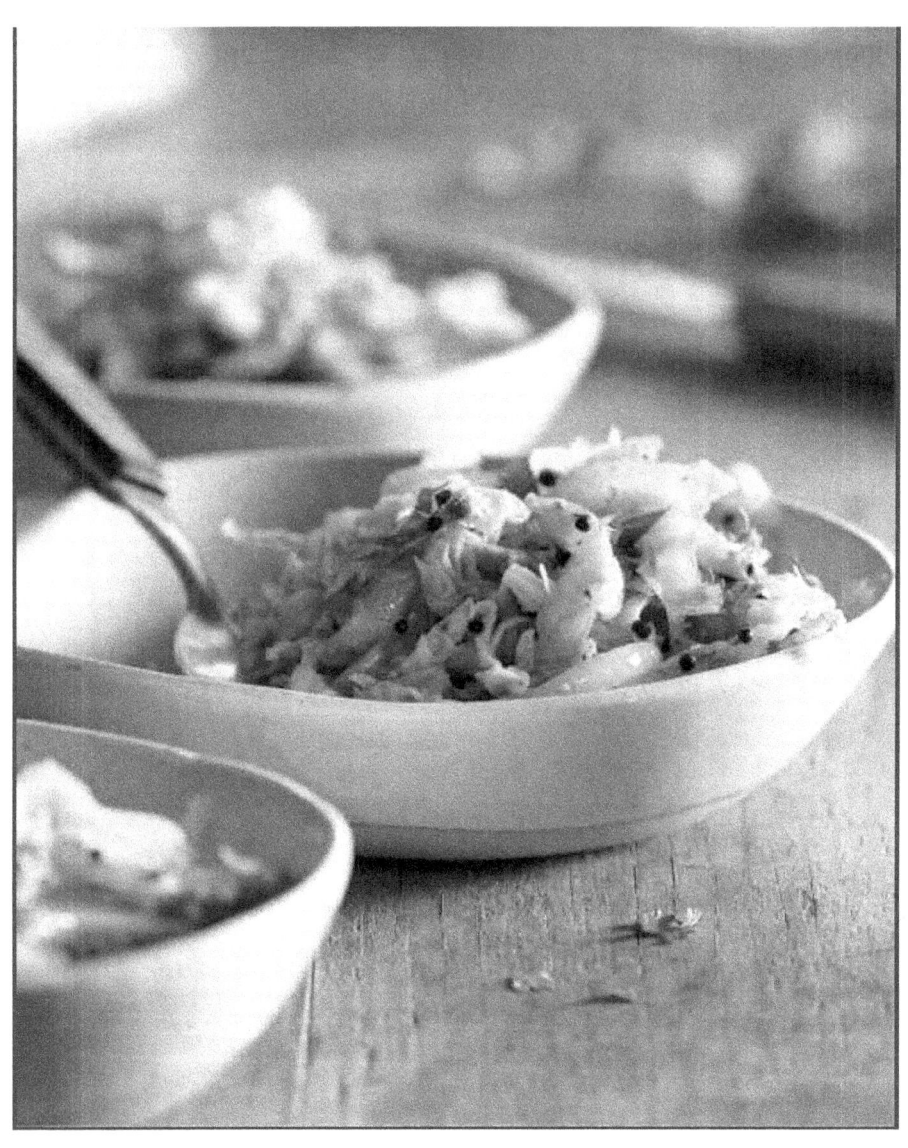

PUNJABI-STYLE SAVOY CABBAGE

PREP: 20 minutes COOK: 25 minutes MAKES: 4 servings PHOTO

IT'S AMAZING WHAT HAPPENS TO A MILDLY-FLAVORED, UNASSUMING CABBAGE WHEN IT'S COOKED WITH GINGER, GARLIC, CHILES, AND INDIAN SPICES. TOASTED MUSTARD, CORIANDER, AND CUMIN SEEDS GIVE THIS DISH BOTH FLAVOR AND CRUNCH. BE FOREWARNED: IT IS HOT! BIRD'S BEAK CHILES ARE SMALL BUT VERY POTENT—AND THE DISH INCLUDES JALAPEÑO TOO. IF YOU PREFER LESS HEAT, JUST USE THE JALAPEÑO.

1 2-inch knob fresh ginger, peeled and cut into ⅓-inch slices
5 cloves garlic
1 large jalapeño, stemmed, seeded, and halved (see tip)
2 teaspoons no-salt-added garam masala
1 teaspoon ground turmeric
½ cup Chicken Bone Broth (see recipe) or no-salt-added chicken broth
3 tablespoons refined coconut oil
1 tablespoon black mustard seeds
1 teaspoon coriander seeds
1 teaspoon cumin seeds
1 whole bird's beak chile (chile de arbol) (see tip)
1 3-inch cinnamon stick
2 cups thinly sliced yellow onions (about 2 medium)
12 cups thinly sliced, cored savoy cabbage (about 1½ pounds)
½ cup snipped fresh cilantro (optional)

1. In a food processor or blender combine ginger, garlic, jalapeño, garam masala, turmeric, and ¼ cup of the Chicken Bone Broth. Cover and process or blend until smooth; set aside.

2. In an extra-large skillet combine coconut oil, mustard seeds, coriander seeds, cumin seeds, chile, and cinnamon stick. Cook over medium-high heat, shaking pan frequently, for 2 to 3 minutes or until the cinnamon stick unfurls.(Be careful—mustard seeds will pop and spatter as they cook.) Add onions; cook and stir for 5 to 6 minutes or until onions are lightly browned. Add ginger mixture. Cook, for 6 to 8 minutes or until mixture is nicely caramelized, stirring often.

3. Add cabbage and the remaining Chicken Bone Broth; mix well. Cover and cook about 15 minutes or until cabbage is tender, stirring twice. Uncover skillet. Cook and stir for 6 to 7 minutes or until cabbage is lightly browned and excess Chicken Bone Broth evaporates.

4. Remove and discard cinnamon stick and chile. If desired, sprinkle with cilantro.

CINNAMON-ROASTED BUTTERNUT SQUASH

PREP: 20 minutes ROAST: 30 minutes MAKES: 4 to 6 servings

A DASH OF CAYENNE PEPPER GIVES THESE SWEET ROASTED CUBES OF SQUASH JUST A HINT OF HEAT. IT'S EASILY LEFT OUT IF YOU PREFER. SERVE THIS SIMPLE SIDE WITH ROAST PORK OR PORK CHOPS.

1 butternut squash (about 2 pounds), peeled, seeded, and cut into ¾-inch cubes
2 tablespoons olive oil
½ teaspoon ground cinnamon
¼ teaspoon black pepper
⅛ teaspoon cayenne pepper

1. Preheat oven to 400°F. In a large bowl toss squash with olive oil, cinnamon, black pepper, and cayenne pepper. Line a large rimmed baking sheet with parchment paper. Spread squash in a single layer on the baking sheet.

2. Roast for 30 to 35 minutes or until squash is tender and browned on edges, stirring once or twice.

BROILED ASPARAGUS WITH SIEVED EGG AND PECANS

START TO FINISH: 15 minutes MAKES: 4 servings

THIS IS A TAKE ON A CLASSIC FRENCH VEGETABLE DISH CALLED ASPARAGUS MIMOSA—SO CALLED BECAUSE THE GREEN, WHITE, AND YELLOW OF THE FINISHED DISH LOOKS LIKE A FLOWER OF THE SAME NAME.

1 pound fresh asparagus, trimmed
5 tablespoons Roasted Garlic Vinaigrette (see recipe)
1 hard-cooked egg, peeled
3 tablespoons chopped pecans, toasted (see tip)
Freshly ground black pepper

1. Position oven rack 4 inches from heating element; preheat broiler to high.

2. Spread asparagus spears on a baking sheet. Drizzle with 2 tablespoons of the Roasted Garlic Vinaigrette. Using your hands, roll asparagus to coat with vinaigrette. Broil for 3 to 5 minutes or until blistered and tender, turning asparagus after every minute. Transfer to a serving platter.

3. Cut the egg in half; press egg through a sieve over the asparagus. (You can also grate the egg using the large holes of a box grater.) Drizzle asparagus and egg with the remaining 3 tablespoons Roasted Garlic Vinaigrette. Top with pecans and sprinkle with pepper.

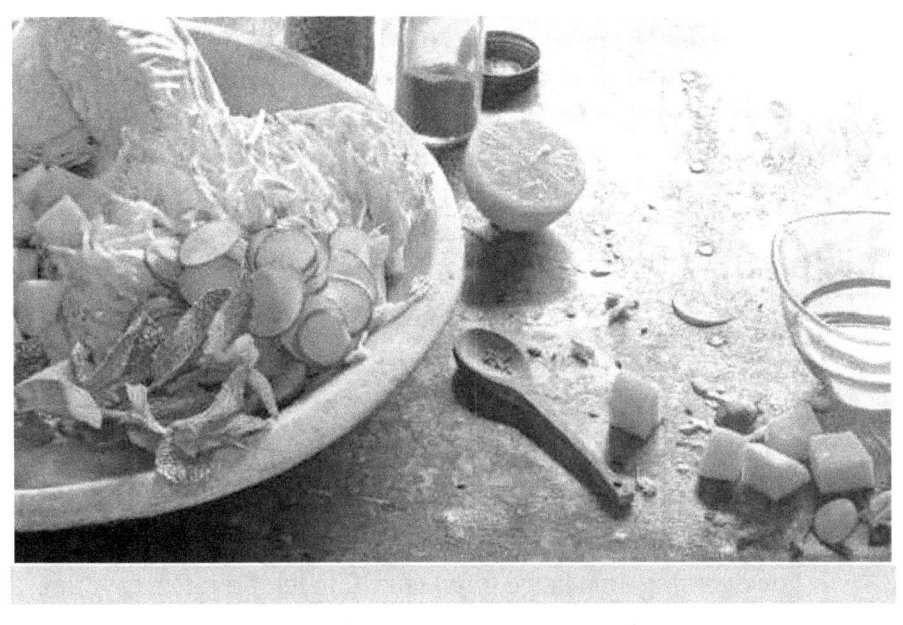

CRUNCHY CABBAGE SLAW WITH RADISHES, MANGO, AND MINT

START TO FINISH: 20 minutes MAKES: 6 servings PHOTO

3 tablespoons fresh lemon juice
¼ teaspoon cayenne pepper
¼ teaspoon ground cumin
¼ cup olive oil
4 cups shredded cabbage
1½ cups very thinly sliced radishes
1 cup cubed ripe mango
½ cup bias-sliced scallions
⅓ cup chopped fresh mint

1. For dressing, in a large bowl combine lemon juice, cayenne pepper, and ground cumin. Whisk in olive oil in a thin stream.

2. Add cabbage, radishes, mango, scallions, and mint to dressing in bowl. Toss well to combine.

ROASTED CABBAGE ROUNDS WITH CARAWAY AND LEMON

PREP: 10 minutes ROAST: 30 minutes MAKES: 4 to 6 servings

3 tablespoons olive oil
1 medium head cabbage, cut into 1-inch-thick rounds
2 teaspoons Dijon-Style Mustard (see recipe)
1 teaspoon finely shredded lemon peel
¼ teaspoon black pepper
1 teaspoon caraway seeds
Lemon wedges

1. Preheat oven to 400°F. Brush a large rimmed baking sheet with 1 tablespoon of the olive oil. Arrange cabbage rounds on the baking sheet; set aside.

2. In a small bowl whisk together the remaining 2 tablespoons olive oil, Dijon-Style Mustard, and lemon peel. Brush over cabbage rounds on baking sheet, making sure mustard and lemon peel are evenly distributed. Sprinkle with pepper and caraway seeds.

3. Roast for 30 to 35 minutes or until cabbage is tender and edges are golden brown. Serve with lemon wedges to squeeze over cabbage.

ROASTED CABBAGE WITH ORANGE-BALSAMIC DRIZZLE

PREP: 15 minutes ROAST: 30 minutes MAKES: 4 servings

3 tablespoons olive oil
1 small head cabbage, cored and cut into 8 wedges
½ teaspoon black pepper
⅓ cup balsamic vinegar
2 teaspoons finely shredded orange peel

1. Preheat oven to 450°F. Brush a large rimmed baking sheet with 1 tablespoon of the olive oil. Arrange cabbage wedges on the baking sheet. Brush cabbage with the remaining 2 tablespoons olive oil and sprinkle with pepper.

2. Roast cabbage for 15 minutes. Turn cabbage wedges over; roast about 15 minutes more or until cabbage is tender and edges are golden brown.

3. In a small saucepan combine the balsamic vinegar and orange peel. Bring to boiling over medium heat; reduce. Simmer, uncovered, about 4 minutes or until reduced by half. Drizzle over roasted cabbage wedges; serve immediately.

BRAISED CABBAGE WITH CREAMY DILL SAUCE AND TOASTED WALNUTS

PREP: 20 minutes COOK: 40 minutes MAKES: 6 servings

3 tablespoons olive oil
1 shallot, finely chopped
1 small head green cabbage, cut into 6 wedges
½ teaspoon black pepper
1 cup Chicken Bone Broth (see recipe) or no-salt-added chicken broth
¾ cup Cashew Cream (see recipe)
4 teaspoons finely shredded lemon peel
4 teaspoons snipped fresh dill
1 tablespoon finely chopped scallions
¼ cup chopped walnuts, toasted (see tip)

1. In an extra-large skillet heat olive oil over medium-high heat. Add shallot; cook for 2 to 3 minutes or until tender and lightly browned. Add cabbage wedges to skillet. Cook, uncovered, for 10 minutes or until lightly browned on each side, turning once halfway through cooking. Sprinkle with pepper.

2. Add Chicken Bone Broth to skillet. Bring to boiling; reduce heat. Cover and simmer for 25 to 30 minutes or until cabbage is tender.

3. Meanwhile, for Creamy Dill Sauce, in a small bowl stir together Cashew Cream, lemon peel, dill, and scallions.

4. To serve, transfer cabbage wedges to serving plates; drizzle with pan juices. Top with dill sauce and sprinkle with toasted walnuts.

SAUTÉED GREEN CABBAGE WITH TOASTED SESAME SEEDS

PREP: 20 minutes COOK: 19 minutes MAKES: 4 servings

2 tablespoons sesame seeds
2 tablespoons refined coconut oil
1 medium onion, thinly sliced
1 medium tomato, chopped
1 tablespoon minced fresh ginger
3 cloves garlic, minced
¼ teaspoon crushed red pepper
½ of a 3- to 3½-pound head green cabbage, cored and very thinly sliced

1. In an extra-large dry skillet toast sesame seeds over medium heat for 3 to 4 minutes or until golden brown, stirring almost constantly. Transfer seeds to a smal bowl and cool completely. Transfer seeds to a clean spice or coffee grinder; pulse to grind coarsely. Set ground sesame seeds aside.

2. Meanwhile, in the same extra-large skillet heat coconut oil over medium-high heat. Add onion; cook about 2 minutes or just until slightly soft. Stir in tomato, ginger, garlic, and crushed red pepper. Cook and stir for 2 minutes more.

3. Add sliced cabbage to tomato mixture in skillet. Toss with tongs to combine. Cook for 12 to 14 minutes or until cabbage is tender and just begins to brown, stirring occasionally. Add ground sesame seeds; stir well to combine. Serve immediately.

www.ingramcontent.com/pod-product-compliance
Lightning Source LLC
Chambersburg PA
CBHW071822080526
44589CB00012B/886